Ultrasound Mammography

B.-J. Hackelöer V. Duda G. Lauth

Ultrasound Mammography

Methods, Results, Diagnostic Strategies

With the Collaboration of Jack Jellins
Foreword by Elizabeth Kelly-Fry

With 186 Illustrations in 404 Parts, 6 in Full Color

Springer-Verlag
New York Berlin Heidelberg
London Paris Tokyo

B.-JOACHIM HACKELÖER, M.D.
Professor of Obstetrics and Gynecology, University of Marburg, Marburg; Professor of Obstetrics and Gynecology, University of Hamburg, Hamburg, Federal Republic of Germany

VOLKER DUDA, M.D.
Department of Obstetrics and Gynecology, University of Marburg, Marburg, Federal Republic of Germany

GÜNTHER LAUTH, M.D.
Director, Department of Gynecologic Radiology, University of Marburg, Marburg, Federal Republic of Germany

JACK JELLINS, Ph.D., FAIUM
Head, Ultrasonic Imaging, Ultrasonics Institute, Chatswood, NSW, Australia

Translation by T.C. TELGER

Translation and revision of *Ultraschall-Mammographie: Methoden, Ergebnisse, diagnostische Strategien,* © Springer-Verlag, Berlin, 1986.

Library of Congress Cataloging-in-Publication Data
Hackelöer, B.-J. (Bernhard-Joachim), 1945–
[Ultraschall-Mammographie. English]
Ultrasound mammography : methods, results, diagnostic strategies / B.-J. Hackelöer, V. Duda, G. Lauth, with the collaboration of Jack Jellins ; foreword by Elizabeth Kelly-Fry ; [translation by T.C. Telger.]
p. cm.
Translation and revision of: Ultraschall-Mammographie.
Includes bibliography and index.
1. Breast—Ultrasonic imaging. 2. Breast—Diseases—Diagnosis I. Duda, V. (Volker) II. Lauth, Günther. III. Jellins, Jack. IV. Title.
[DNLM: 1. Mammography. 2. Ultrasonic Diagnosis. WP 815 H118u]
RG493.5.U47H3313 1988
618.1'907543—dc19
DNLM/DLC 88-6419

Printed on acid-free paper.

Softcover reprint of the hardcover 1st edition 1989

Typeset by Publishers Service, Bozeman, Montana.

9 8 7 6 5 4 3 2 1

ISBN-13: 978-1-4612-8116-0 e-ISBN-13: 978-1-4612-3476-0
DOI: 10.1007/978-1-4612-3476-0

To our wives

Foreword

For most areas of medical ultrasound, textbooks that provide physicians with detailed, practical information are readily available. Unfortunately, for the field of ultrasound mammography, such texts are few in number, in comparison to the number available for other fields of medical ultrasound. This textbook by Drs. Hackelöer, Duda, and Lauth fills this gap by presenting a clear overview of the usefulness and limitations of ultrasound mammography.

Information based on clinical experiences with various types of automated and real-time instrumentation is presented in a manner that allows physicians to make their own judgments regarding the diagnostic capabilities of ultrasound mammography. It also provides specific information on techniques required to obtain useful diagnostic data. Examples of the many possible image variations of specific breast pathologies are presented.

The advantages of recent real-time systems, when used with a stand-off, are clearly outlined. The authors do not belabor the philosophical dilemma of which system, an automated or a real-time, is best suited for ultrasound mammography. They simply present the information they have gained in their use of both of these systems and indicate that, in the future, a combination of automated and real-time would be the most valuable for the physician.

Research studies that may be valuable but, as yet, have not been brought into routine clinical application are not included in this text. One exception is a contribution by Dr. Jack Jellins, of the Ultrasonics Institute in Australia, on the use of Doppler for detection of breast malignancies. His chapter allows readers to evaluate the current status of this modality and thus make a judgment whether it is currently appropriate for clinical application.

Drs. Hackelöer, Duda, and Lauth are physicians who are concerned about the increasing incidence of breast cancer. Their textbook reflects this concern and presents practical information to other physicians about the extent to which ultrasound mammography, when used in conjunction with X-ray mammography, may provide better detection and diagnosis of benign and malignant breast masses.

Elizabeth Kelly-Fry
Department of Radiology
Indiana University School of Medicine
Indianapolis, Indiana

Preface

This book is the product of years of fruitful collaboration between the Ultrasound Department and the Radiology Department of the Marburg University Women's Hospital. Therapeutic experience at our institute, close contact with the Pathology Department, and an ongoing discussion of the results have enabled us to achieve an optimum combination of measures for the detection and diagnosis of breast disease.

We have combined breast sonography and X-ray mammography since the advent of easy-to-handle real-time scanners, which we have used since 1975 as a guide for needle aspirations and biopsies. The technique of breast thermography also has been practiced and advanced at our center over the last decade.

Since 1979, series of trials have been conducted with an automated whole-breast immersion scanner that have enabled us to characterize the sonographic anatomy of the breast in detail and determine the place of breast ultrasound relative to other modalities. During this time, we have maintained close contact with the principal research groups in Australia, Japan, and the United States.

Experience with the immersion scanner has enabled us, in the last two to three years, to return to the use of commercially available real-time scanners, with and without water-path coupling. Today sonography has become a routine part of every breast examination conducted at our center.

Diagnostic ultrasound has assumed an established place in breast diagnosis. Technical advances (computed sonography) have even made it possible to detect microcalcifications, suggesting that ultrasound may have potential value as a screening tool for breast cancer.

In this book we present a practical model for optimizing the approach to the detection and diagnosis of breast disease.

In response to the growing interest in breast ultrasound, we have created a richly illustrated text that addresses the role of the modality in breast diagnosis as well as the practical concerns of those who select and operate ultrasound instrumentation.

We are particularly indebted to Prof. Dr. R. Buchholz and the P.E. Kempkes Foundation for making our research possible, and to Prof. Dr. K.-D. Schulz for his additional support. We also express thanks to our colleagues and co-workers at the Ultrasound and Radiology Departments and to the Photographic Laboratory under the direction of Mrs. Wenz.

B.-J. Hackelöer
V. Duda
G. Lauth

Contents

1
Basic Technical and Methodologic Aspects of Breast Sonography

Introduction

In 1952 Wild and Reid performed the initial studies that laid the groundwork for the development of breast sonography. The Japanese groups of Wagai and Kobayashi and the Australian groups of Kossoff and Jellins published the first clinically important results in the early 1970s. Their work stimulated a widespread implementation and refinement of breast sonography using real-time instrumentation. Today, computer-controlled systems have given ultrasound an established place in the diagnosis of breast diseases and have made it competitive with other noninvasive modalities.

From the outset, breast ultrasound was plagued by problems of orientation and the lack of a homogenous parenchymal structure, and even today X-ray mammography is considered to be the mainstay of breast imaging. On closer analysis, we find that this is based largely on the ability of radiomammography to detect microcalcifications and on its value as a screening device.

But experience in recent years has shown that breast sonography is already the primary modality for examinations of the dense breast and for the evaluation of benign disorders. With further improvements in resolution over the depth and width of the image field, sonography may even become the primary imaging modality in general for breast examinations. Computerization of the signal transmission and processing functions has led to a new generation of scanners that promise new results in the structural evaluation of parenchymatous organs. Initial trials with one such instrument (the Acuson) have already demonstrated a capability for the reproducible imaging of breast microcalcifications (see Chap. 5).

The potential of sonography in routine screening remains unclear. Even computerization does not change one basic aspect of the ultrasound examination—the need to obtain multiple, thin, cross-sectional image "slices" that the examiner must then assemble into a total picture in order to make a diagnosis. The experience of the examiner is decisive in this regard—it is not enough to produce technically flawless images. This fact distinguishes sonography from other methods that produce summation images. It also greatly limits the use of technical aids like those employed in X-ray mammography. The problem is that generally we are unable to specify accurately reproducible scanning planes in the breast. An exception is automated immersion scanning, in which planes can be defined using the nipple as a reference. If the use of ultrasound is confined to the investigation of palpable breast masses, it is not essential that scanning planes be specified. But if the method is to be applied for the screening or early detection of breast cancer, the scanning protocol must be clearly and unambiguously defined.

A major goal of this book is to offer guidelines that will enable diagnostic breast ultrasound to be applied rationally and to its full potential. Medically and forensically, of course, diagnostic workup still requires that other methods and modalities be employed also and that breast sonography be performed only by properly trained and experienced physicians.

Fundamentals of the Examination Technique

In recent years ultrasound has gained an established place in the evaluation of breast disease (Fig. 1.1). A variety of techniques have been used to image the breast with ultrasound. Conventional echography employs a hand-held real-time scanner, with or without water-path coupling (Fig. 1.2). This technique involves some degree of breast compression, depending on the coupling pressure and the individual shape and firmness of the breast. Because the image produced by a hand-held scanner covers only a relatively small sector of the breast, orientation is extremely difficult, if not impossible. It is difficult to reproduce specific planes in follow-up examinations, although some instruments now provide means of documenting the image plane directly on the sonogram (Fig. 1.3). Superficial structures can be imaged more clearly by coupling hand-held instruments to the skin via a water or plastic path, taking care that this does not shift the area of interest out of the focal region of the transducer (Fig. 1.4). The hand-held real-time technique is excellent for the delineation of palpable masses and for guiding and monitoring needle aspirations and biopsies of the breast (Fig. 1.5). With cysts, the success of a sonographically guided aspiration can be confirmed by withdrawing fluid and documenting the collapse of the mass; the aspiration of solid tumors can be monitored by identifying the tip of the needle on the scan. In the latter case it is sufficient to demonstrate the needle tip in a central area of the tumor on a single plane, in contrast to the summation imaging technique of X-ray mammography, where needle placement always must be documented on two planes. The time and monetary costs of the hand-held real-time technique are relatively small.

This contrasts with the automated immersion scanner technique, in which the patient is positioned prone with the breast freely suspended in water (Fig. 1.6). The water tank contains two or more sector transducers (depending on the instrument type) that beam ultrasound into the breast from different directions but on one plane. These scanners can survey the entire breast with serial scans taken at designated intervals on transverse or longitudinal planes. The nipple provides an ideal reference plane for this technique (Fig. 1.7). If necessary, the examiner may additionally take scans on oblique or rotational planes outside the transverse and longitudinal projections. The scans obtained may be simple or compound, depending on the number of transducers activated (Fig. 1.8). Compound scans yield a complex image containing numerous scattered echoes and few if any secondary features. Simple scans contain fewer scatter echoes and their secondary features are easier to evaluate, but there is a danger that lesions may be missed by a beam that penetrates the breast from one direction only. Although compression can be applied in immersion scanners by the use of a plastic band, this appears to be disadvantageous because it pushes the nipple down to skin level and effaces a critical landmark for orientation. A common problem with the immersion technique is lack of correlation with palpable findings. Also, the method is relatively costly and time consuming.

In a technique that is intermediate between the contact and immersion methods, the patient is positioned supine and a water bag containing an automated scanner is placed in contact with the breast that is to be examined. A similar technique can be applied to patients in the sitting position.

The preferred image format for breast sonography is white echoes on a black background. The studies published by Sanders show that substantially fewer echoes are needed to produce a satisfactory image than in the black-on-white format (Fig. 1.9) (Sanders, 1980).

Some systems have the capability of image "post-processing," that is, manipulation of the gray scale to accentuate image details. This can be advantageous in selected cases (Fig. 1.10).

There are various means of documenting breast scans, including the use of instant-image and small-format cameras, multiformat systems, and videotape. Illustrative sonograms should be sufficient for hand-held real-time examinations, but a more thorough and systematic record is preferred for automated scans (Fig. 1.11).

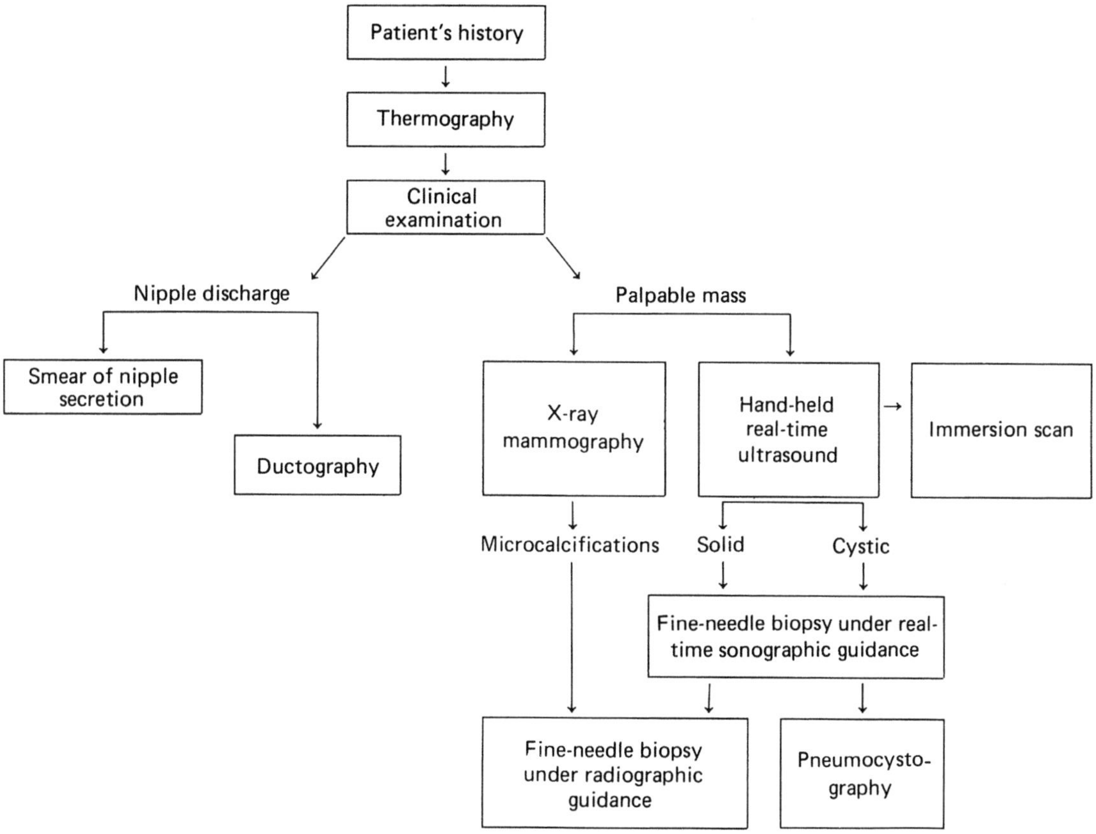

Fig. 1.1. Flowchart for the evaluation of breast disease.

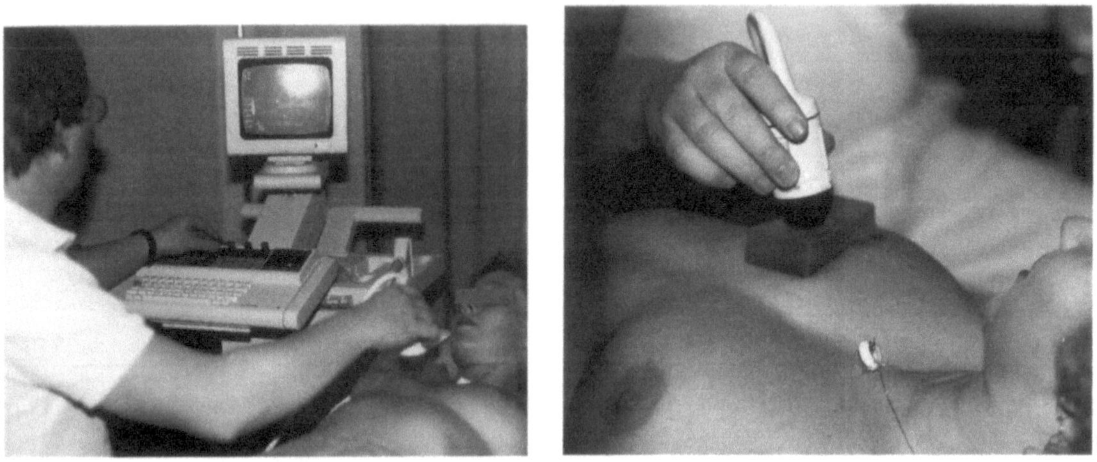

Fig. 1.2a,b. Hand-held real-time breast sonography using a coupling path.

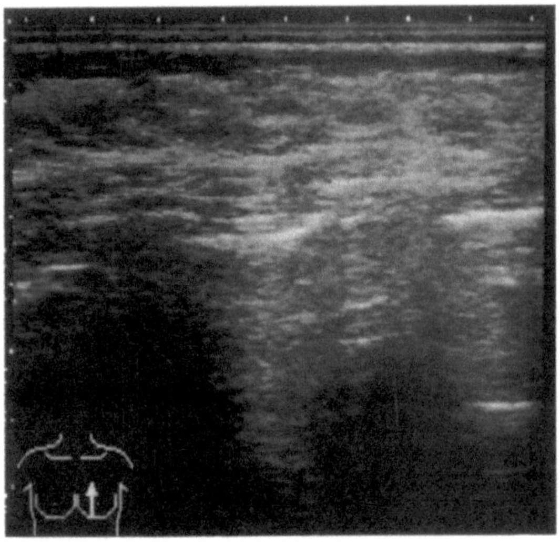

Fig. 1.3. Documentation of the scan plane on a real-time ultrasound instrument

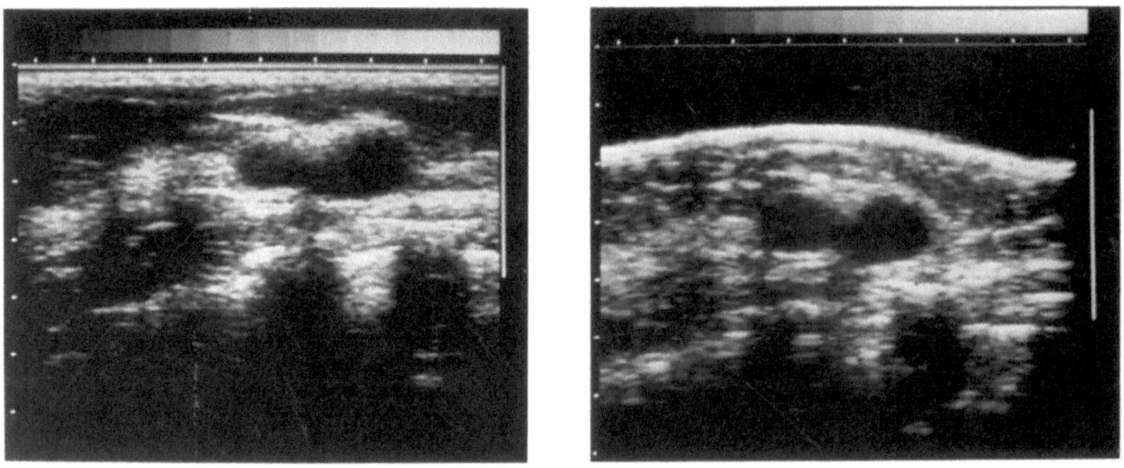

Fig. 1.4a,b. Real-time sonograms of two closely adjacent breast cysts. **a** Without a coupling path. **b** With a "plastic coupling path"

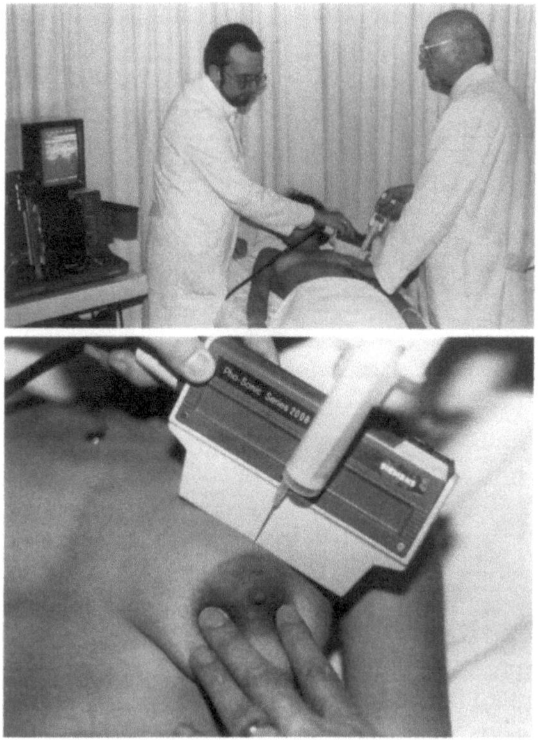

a

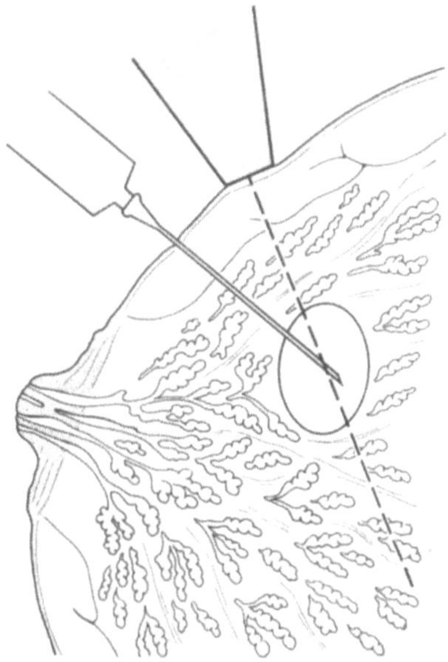

b

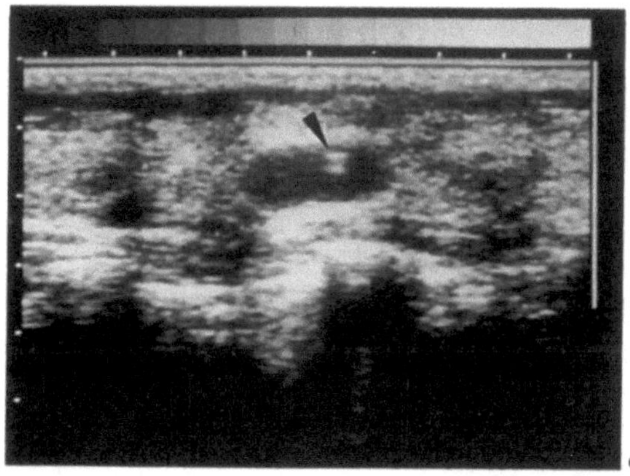

c

Fig. 1.5. Aspiration of the breast. **a** Fine-needle aspiration under sonographic guidance. **b** Transducer placement for ultrasound-guided aspiration of a cyst. **c** Appearance of the needle tip within the cyst

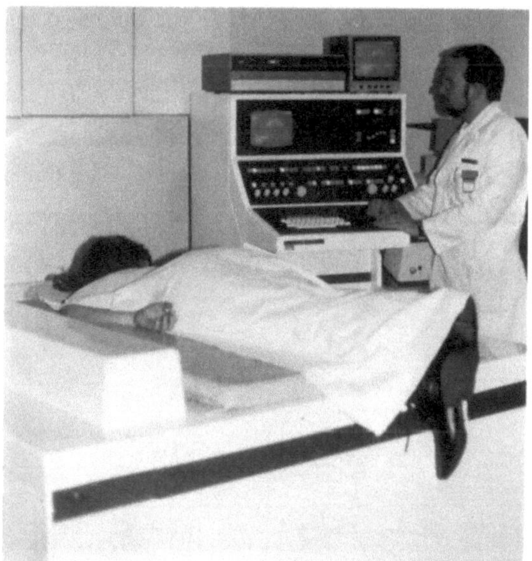

Fig. 1.6. Breast sonography with an immersion scanner

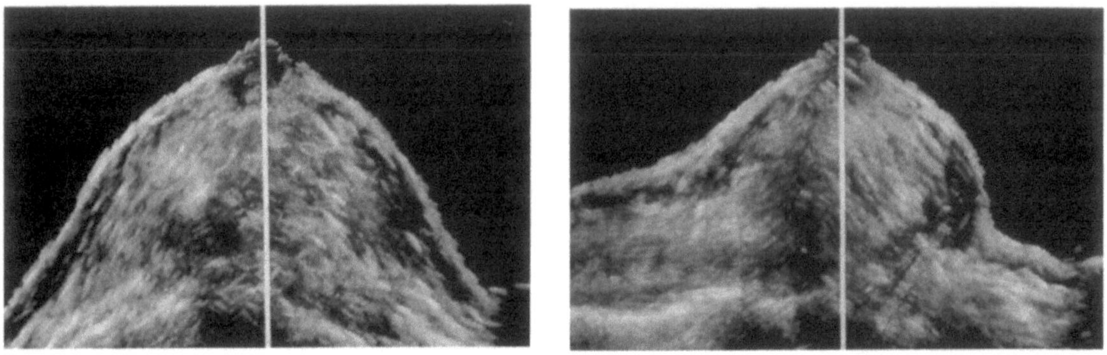

a b

Fig. 1.7a,b. The nipple as a reference point and rotational axis in automated immersion scanning. **a** Transverse scan. **b** Longitudinal scan

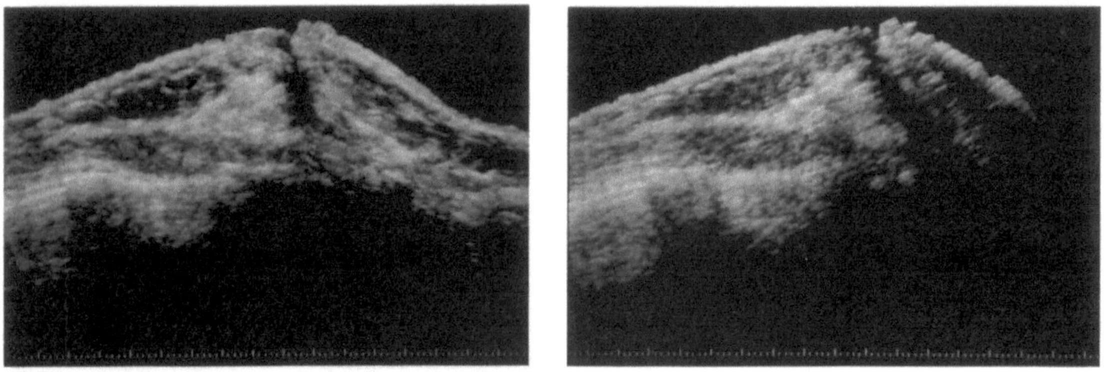

a b

Fig. 1.8. a Compound scan of a centrally located breast carcinoma with ill-defined margins. **b** Simple scan (same plane as in **a**) showing a prominent acoustic shadow behind the mass

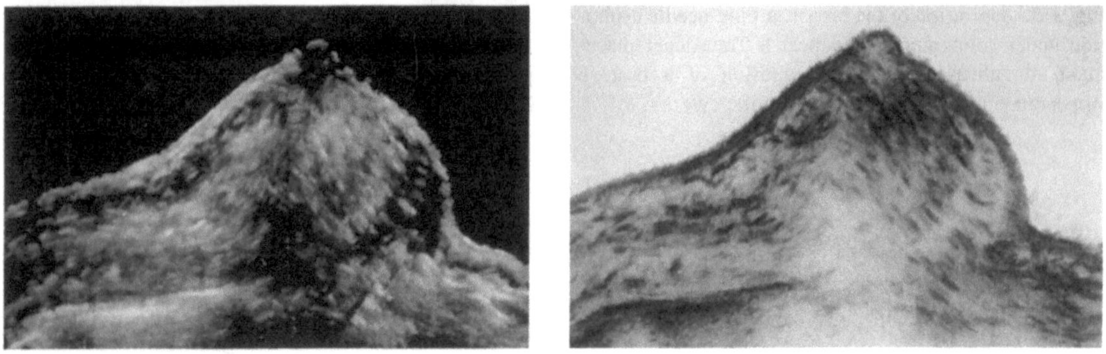

a b

Fig. 1.9a,b. Breast sonograms: **a** White-on-black format. **b** Black-on-white format

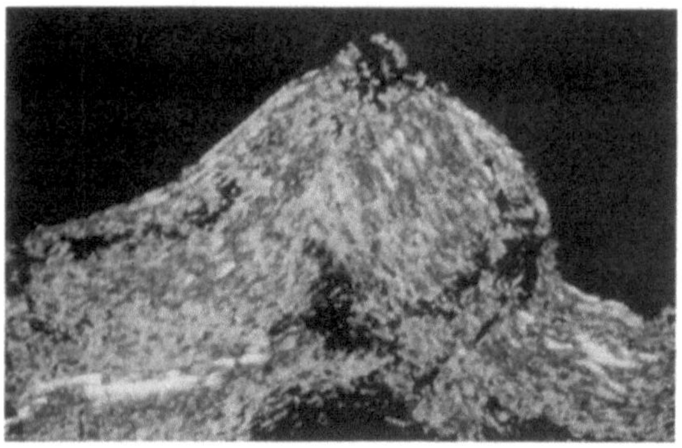

Fig. 1.10. Normal breast sonogram after "postprocessing"
◄

Fig. 1.11. Example of a multiformat image record ►

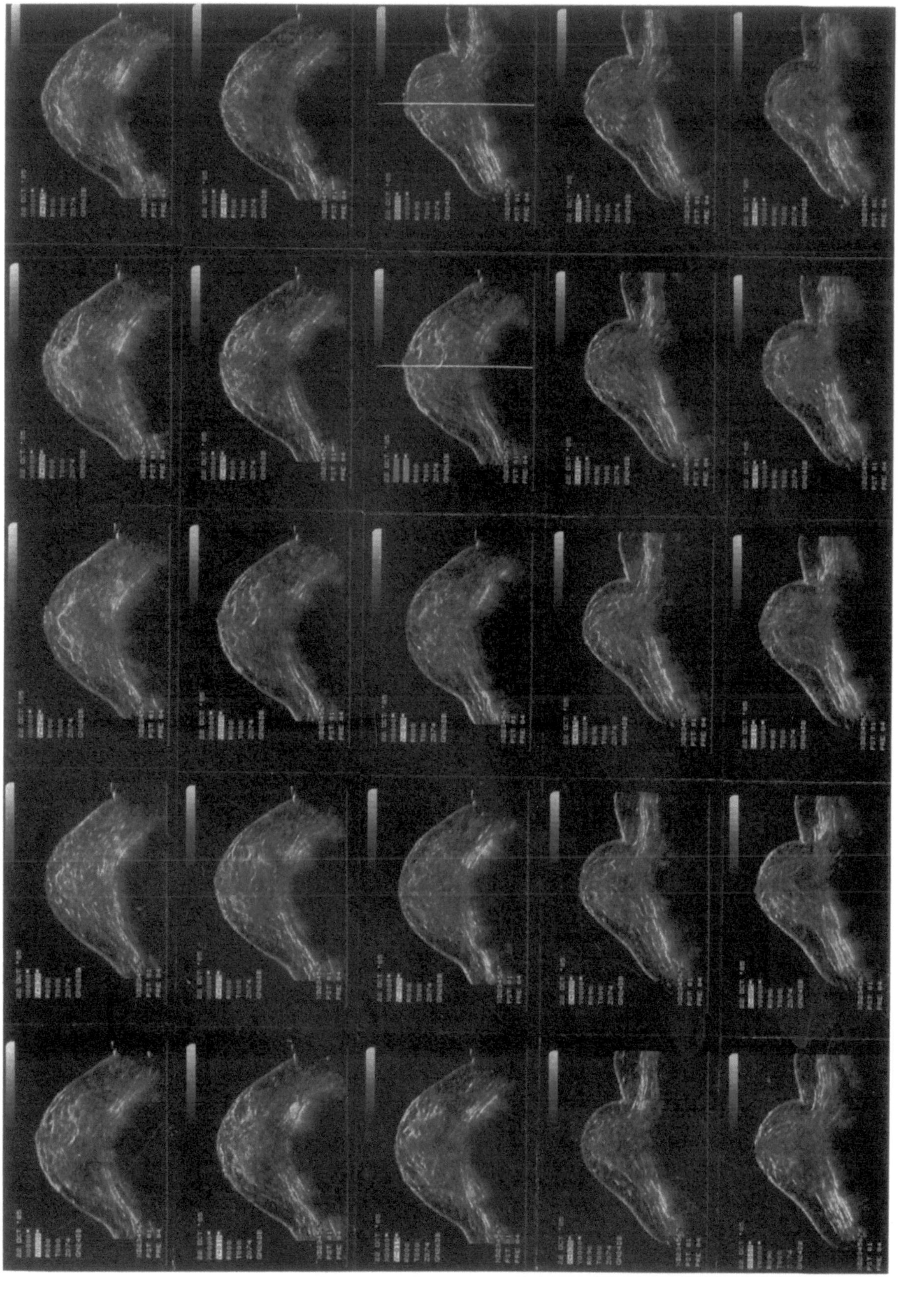

Anatomic Structures and Their Sonographic Correlates

Breast sonograms are indirect anatomic cross sections produced by echoes that form at the interfaces of tissues having different acoustic properties. The basic anatomic structures of the breast produce ultrasound images whose features are easily recognized (Figs. 1.12–1.17; Table 1.1).

Table 1.1. Sonographic correlates of anatomic structures in and around the breast.

Structure	Sonographic features
Nipple	Can be utilized as reference plane; acoustic shadowing of undetermined cause ("nipple shadow") occasionally seen deep to nipple
Skin	Continuous hyperechoic band
Subcutaneous fat layer	More or less strongly defined; hypoechoic
Cooper's ligaments	Extend from base of breast to skin, usually visible as hyperechoic bands in subcutaneous fat
Mammary layer (glandular tissue)	More or less weakly hypoechoic parenchyma containing hyperechoic connective tissue
Milk ducts	Fine, hypoechoic to anechoic, straight or tortuous tubular structures that often dilate on entry into nipple (Fig. 1.14)
Cutaneous veins	Hyperechoic double lines located just beneath skin surface (Fig. 1.15)
Axillary structures (Fig. 1.16)	Occasionally require differentiation from accessory glandular tissue in axillary region (Fig. 1.17)
Chest wall structures	Pectoral fascia, pectoralis, and intercostal muscles, ribs

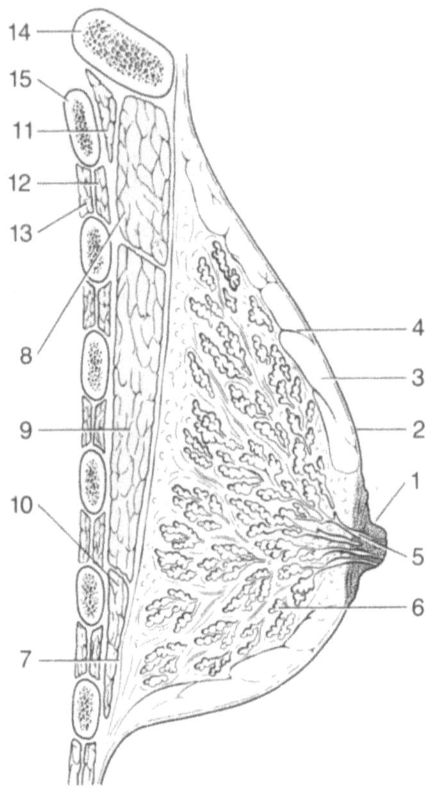

Fig. 1.12. Principal anatomic structures of and around the breast
1 Nipple
2 Skin
3 Subcutaneous fat layer
4 Cooper's ligaments
5 Lactiferous duct, lacteriferous sinus
6 Lobe
7 Pectoral fascia
8 Clavicular part — Pectoralis major muscle
9 Sternocostal part
10 Abdominal part
11 Subclavian muscle
12 External intercostal muscles
13 Internal intercostal muscles
14 Clavicle
15 Ribs

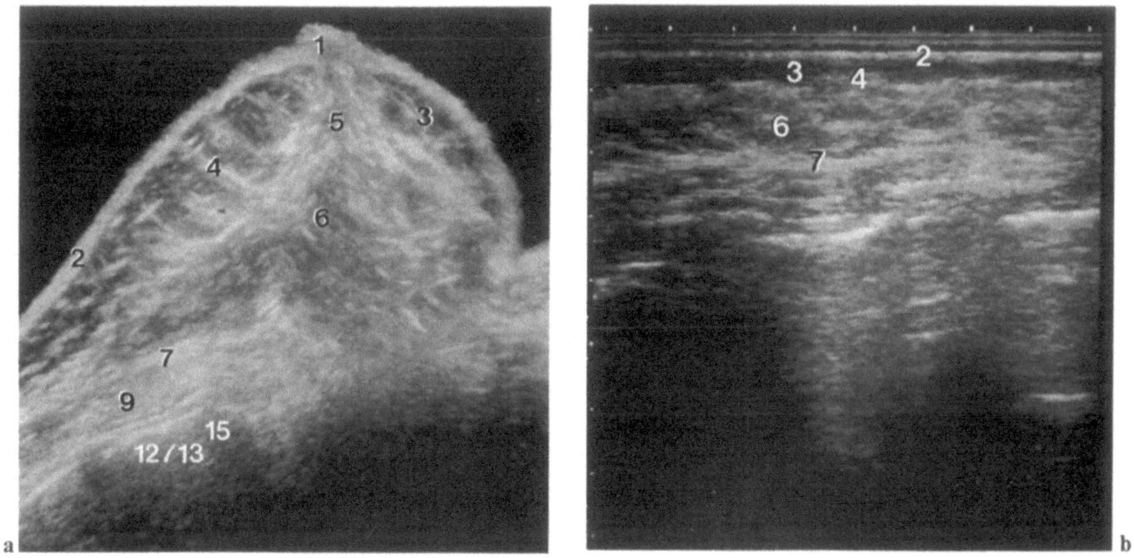

Fig. 1.13a,b. Sonographic appearance of anatomic structures (numbers refer to structures in Fig. 1.12). **a** Immersion scan. **b** Real-time scan

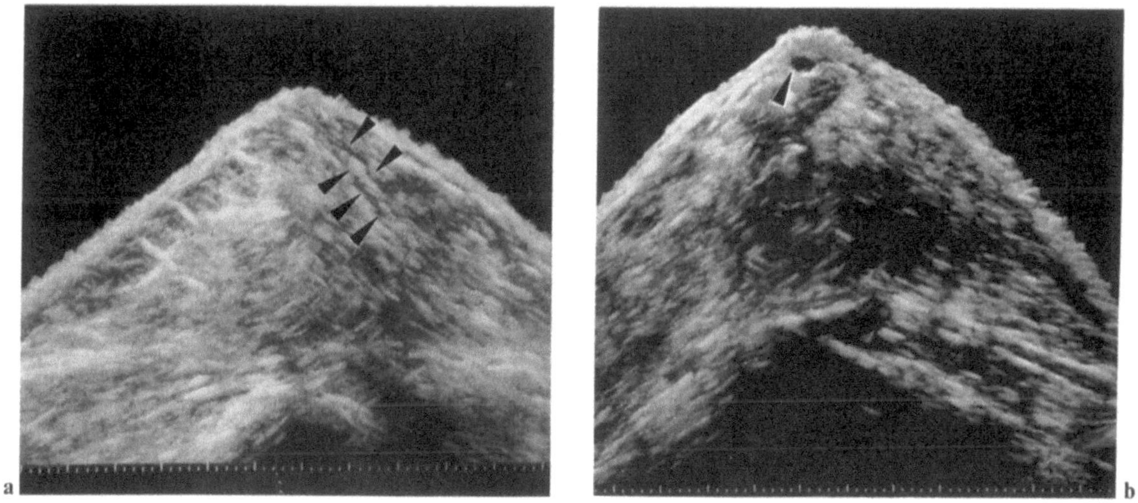

Fig. 1.14. **a** Lactiferous duct. **b** Lactiferous sinus

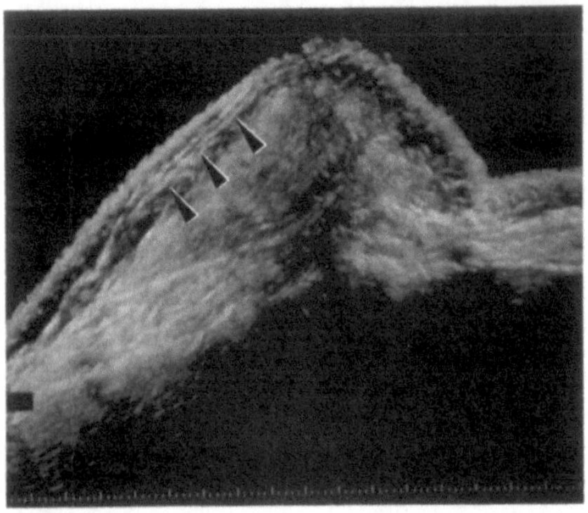

Fig. 1.15. Cutaneous vein

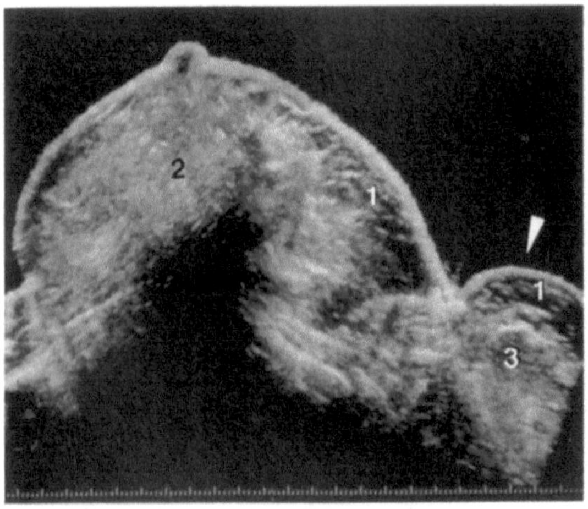

Fig. 1.16. Breast sonogram on a plane traversing the axilla. 1, tissue; 2, glandular tissue; 3, axillary muscles

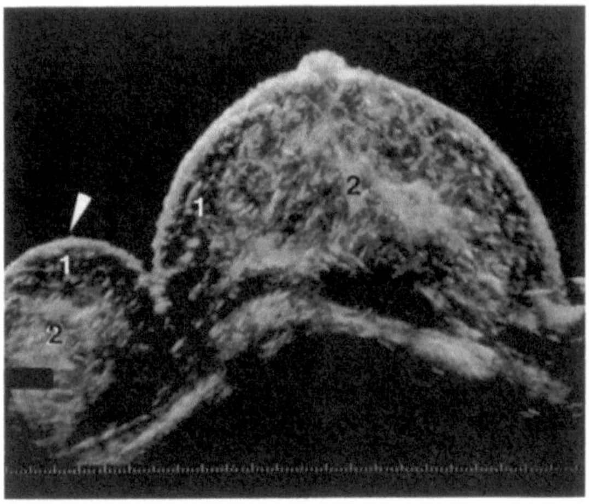

Fig. 1.17. Breast sonogram in the presence of an accessory mammary gland. 1, tissue; 2, glandular tissue

Glandular Tissue

Within the first 3 weeks after birth, the glandular tissue in the newborn's breast enlarges under the influence of residual placental hormones. The milk ducts undergo a cystic dilatation and collect a secretion composed of fat, leukocytes, and desquamated epithelium ("witch's milk").

True maturation of the glandular tissue does not occur until the time of the thelarche, at about 10 to 11 years of age (Fig. 1.18).

After puberty we can distinguish various types of glandular tissue according to the relationship of breast parenchyma to connective tissue and fat (Table 1.2, Figs. 1.19–1.23). We find that the types differ in their accessibility to evaluation with ultrasound, and that all can be correlated with specific age groups or developmental stages in the life of the female (Table 1.3).

Table 1.2. Sonographic breast types and their accessibility to evaluation with ultrasound.

Breast type	Ultrasound evaluation
Dense with strong central absorption (Fig. 1.19)	Breast type of young women; easy to evaluate when compression is applied, but often poorly demonstrated on immersion scans since peripheral and central areas require different time gain compensations for optimum detail
Homogeneously dense (Fig. 1.20)	Breast type of middle-aged women; generally can be easily evaluated
Lactating (Fig. 1.21)	Focal lesions easy to evaluate, but diffuse changes difficult because of prominent duct pattern
Partially involuted (Fig. 1.22)	Breast type of older woman; often difficult to delineate focal lesions in involuted areas; diagnosis may be aided in these cases by breast compression
Involuted (Fig. 1.23)	Breast type of elderly women; hypoechoicity of breast can greatly complicate search for focal lesions

Table 1.3. Frequency and age distribution of sonographic breast types.

Sonographic breast type	Frequency (%) (n=404)	Average age distribution (years)
Dense with strong acoustic absorption	22	<40
Homogeneously dense	38	40–50
Partially involuted	35	50–70
Involuted	5	>70; sometimes seen after mid 20s

Fig. 1.18–1.23. Appearance of the different sonographic breast types on immersion and real-time scans

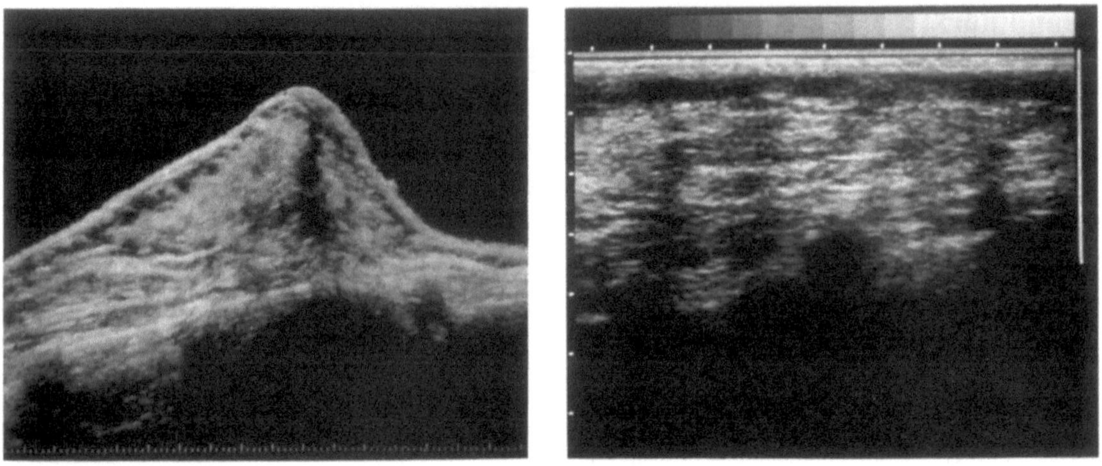

a b

Fig. 1.18a,b. Pubertal breast

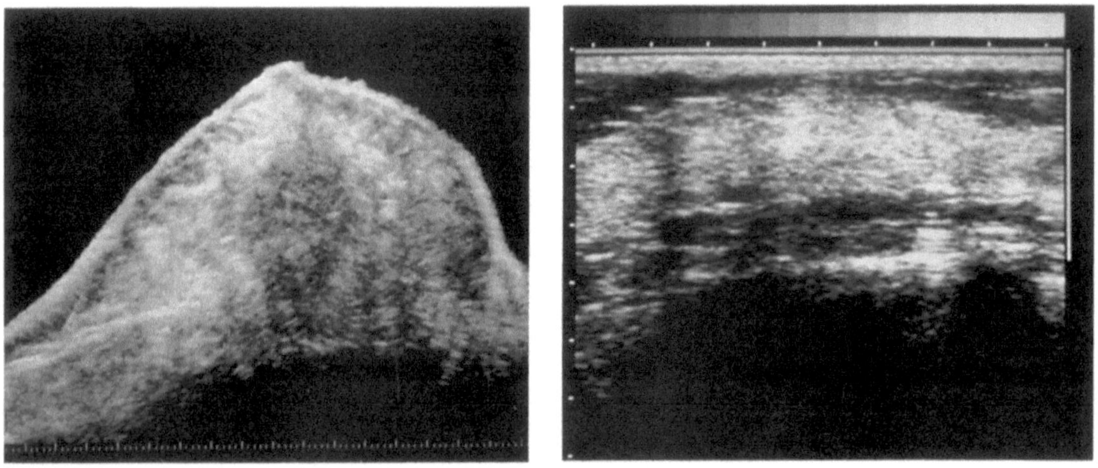

a b

Fig. 1.19a,b. Dense breast with strong central acoustic absorption

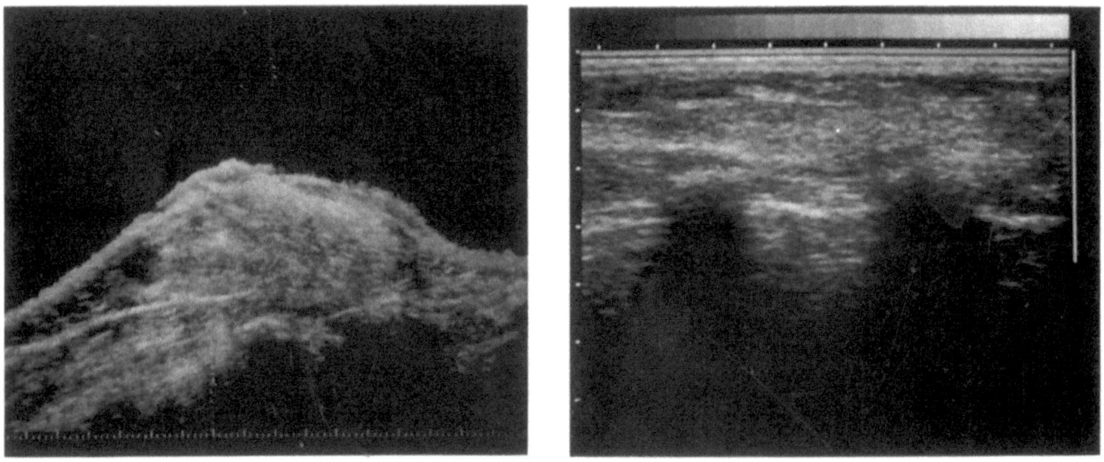

a b

Fig. 1.20a,b. Homogeneously dense breast

a 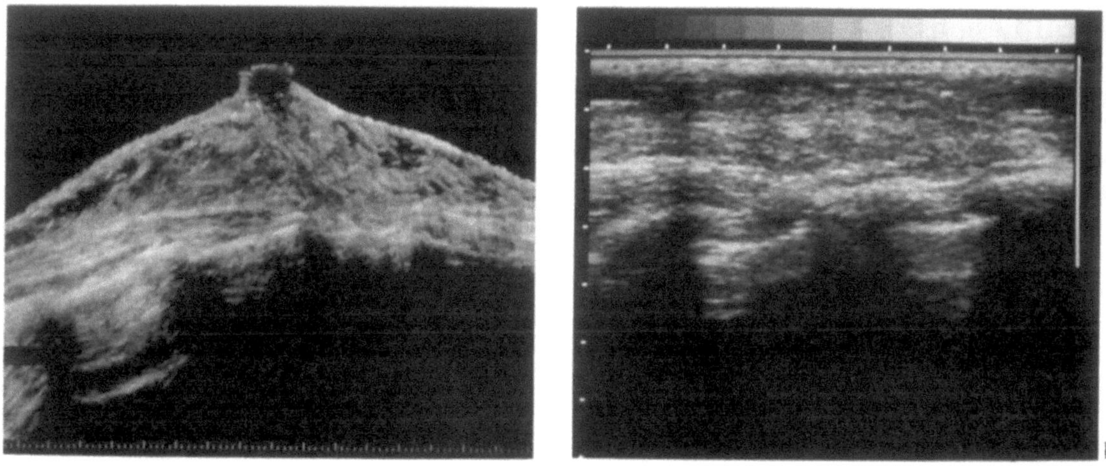 b

Fig. 1.21a,b. Lactating breast

a 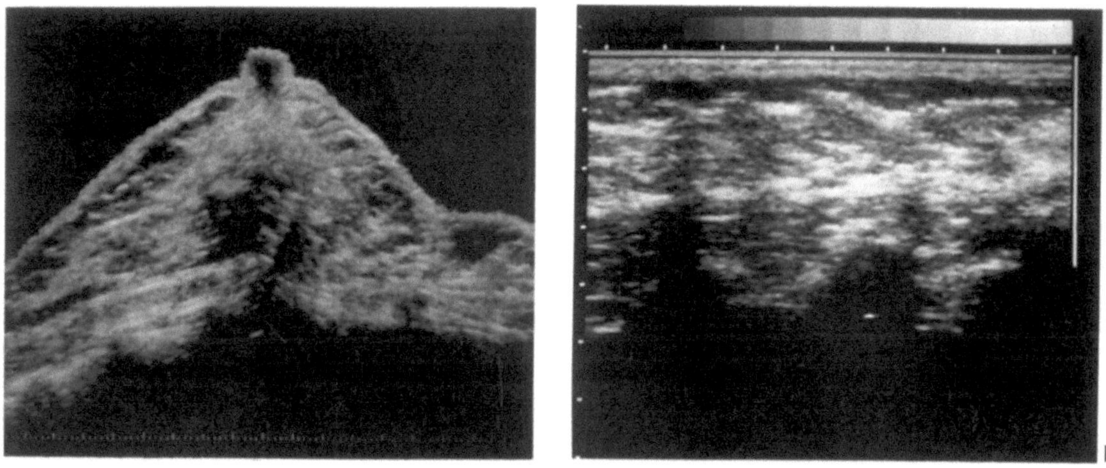 b

Fig. 1.22a,b. Partially involuted breast

a 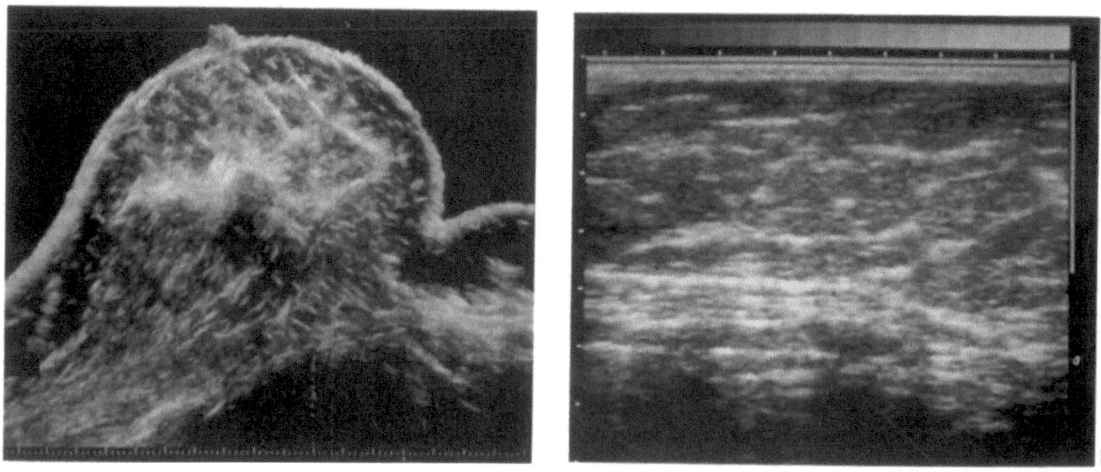 b

Fig. 1.23a,b. Involuted breast

Focal Lesions

For a focal lesion to be clearly delineated with ultrasound, it must lie within the focal region of the transducer (Fig. 1.24), and the time gain compensation (TGC) must be correctly adjusted. The latter can be difficult, because different settings may be needed for different areas of the breast on the same scan (Fig. 1.25). Besides TGC adjustment, optimum imaging requires that the plane be centered on the area of interest rather than being cut peripherally or tangentially (Fig. 1.26). In selected cases, secondary phenomena can be enhanced by the use of a vertical or tangential beam (Fig. 1.27). Hüppe (1982) reported that only 31 of 40 breast carcinomas were clearly delineated with vertical coupling of the transducer, but 38 were clearly shown with tangenetial coupling.

Focal lesions can be characterized sonographically in terms of primary, secondary, and tertiary criteria. Primary criteria relate to the margins and internal echo features of the lesion, while secondary criteria concern phenomena that appear deep to the lesion as a result of its special acoustic properties (enhancement, attenuation, shadowing). Whereas the primary and secondary features characterize a lesion directly, tertiary criteria give indirect evidence of possible pathologic changes in the breast (Table 1.4).

We stipulate that a focal lesion may be identified as such only if it can be demonstrated reproducibly and on two different planes of examination.

Table 1.4. Interpretive criteria for pathologic findings in breast sonograms.

Criterion	Pathologic findings
Primary	Margins [smooth/halo/partly smooth/ill-defined/broom straws (hyperechoic)/fir-tree pattern (hypoechoic)] Internal echoes (structure: regular/irregular/weak; distribution: uniform/non-uniform; hyperechoic areas/anechoic areas)
Secondary	Acoustic enhancement (behind entire lesion/behind portions of lesion) Lateral shadowing (only with smooth-margined lesion or halo) Central shadowing (behind entire lesion/behind portions of lesion/on one plane only/on both planes)
Tertiary	Skin changes (bulging/flattening/retraction/hypoechoic double line of skin thickening/disruption) Disruption of pectoral fascia Axillary lymph nodes Findings suspicious for metastasis on hepatic sonogram

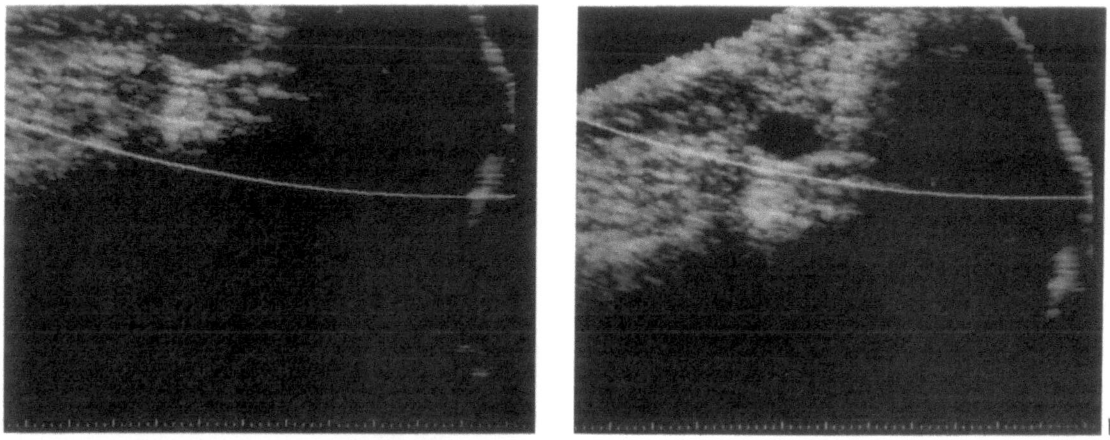

a b

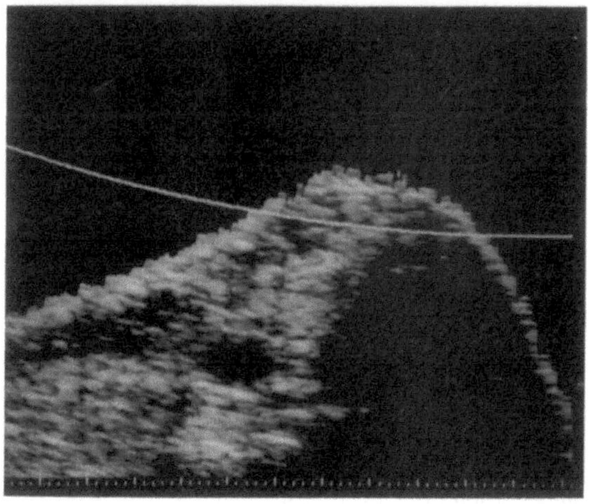

c

Fig. 1.24a-c. Image changes produced by shifting the focal region. **a** The anechoic interior of the cystic mass, **b** its smooth margins, and **c** its posterior enhancement are clearly appreciated only when the mass lies directly within the focal region (indicated by the superimposed arc)

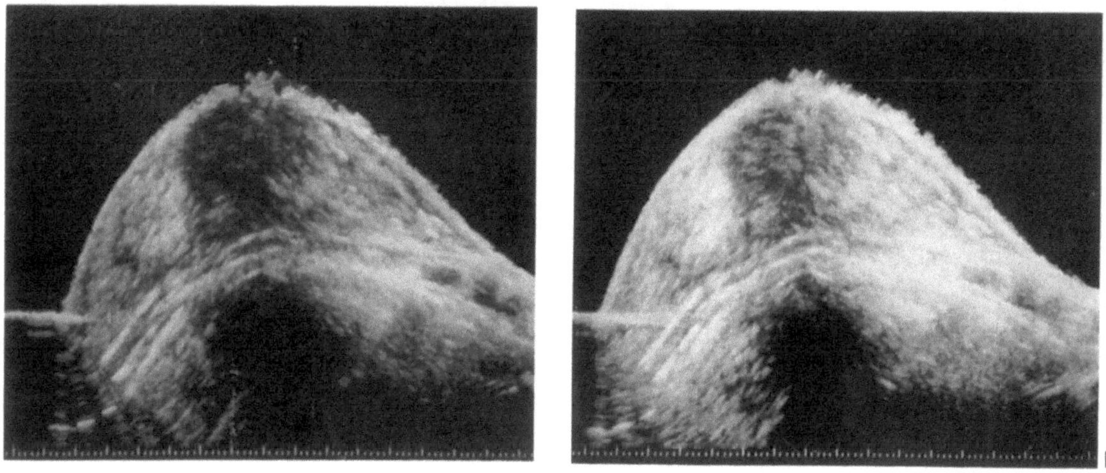

a b

Fig. 1.25a,b. Imaging problems in a breast with very strong central acoustic absorption. **a** The peripheral parts of the mammary layer are well visualized, but the center cannot be evaluated. **b** The center is clearly depicted, but the periphery is washed out.

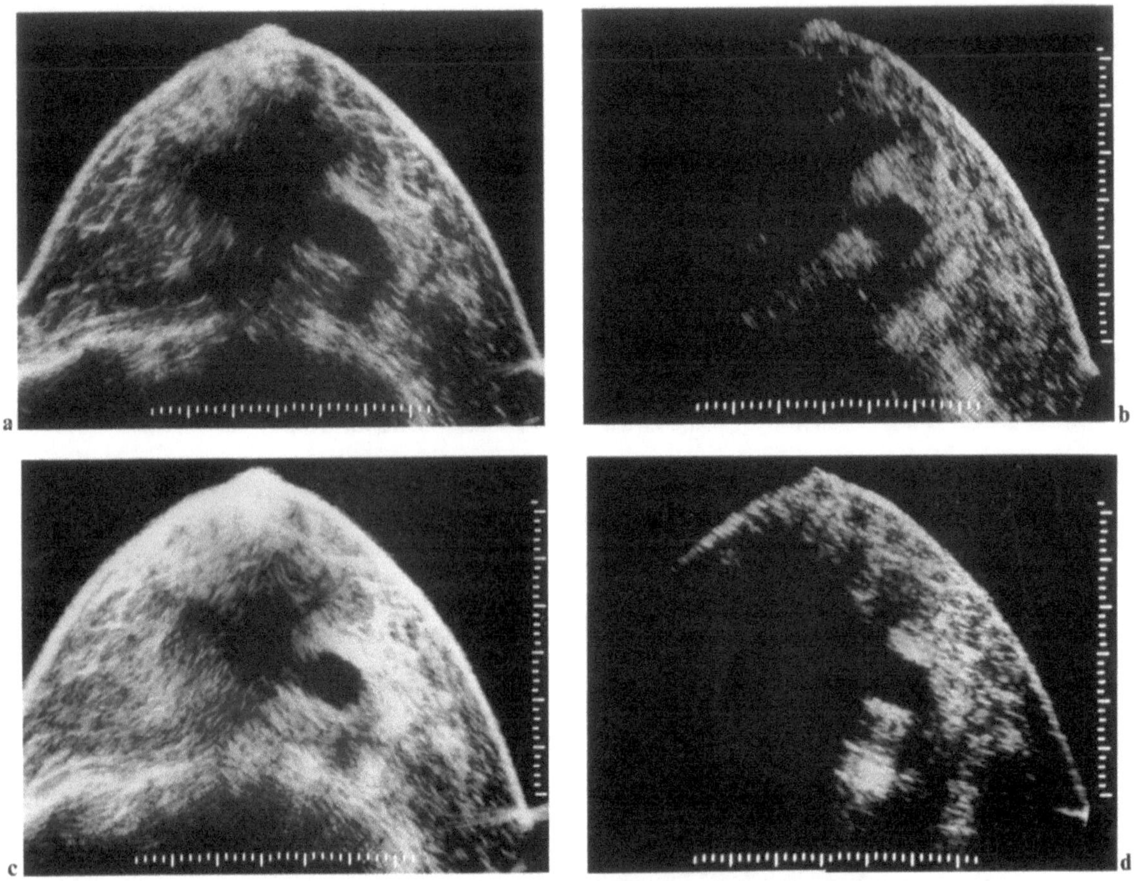

Fig. 1.26a-d. Dependence of image quality on time gain compensation (TGC) and beam angle. **a** TGC is poorly adjusted. **b** Beam angle is too tangential. **c** TGC is well adjusted. **d** Beam angle is correct

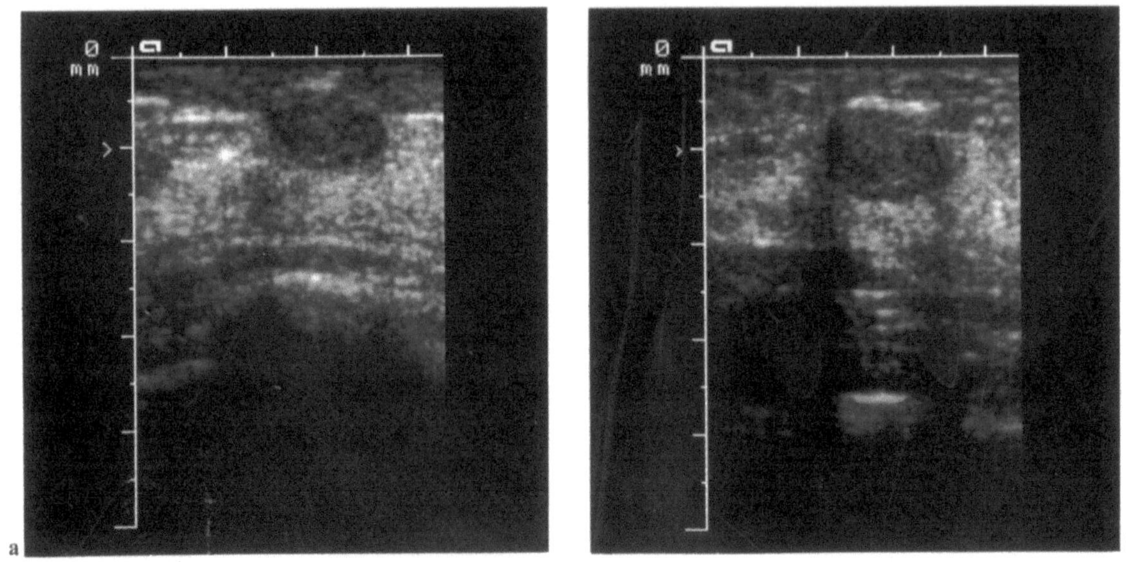

Fig. 1.27. Effect of transducer coupling technique: **a** Vertical coupling produces a satisfactory image of the focal lesion (fibroadenoma). **b** With tangential coupling, the lateral and halo shadowing around the same lesion are more clearly demonstrated

Bibliography

Baum, G. (1983). A comparison of the performance of commercial ultrasound breast scanners versus a laboratory instrument. *Jounal of Clinical Ultrasound 11*:405-413.

Duda, V. (1982). Ultraschall-Mammographie: Das sonographische Erscheinungsbild anatomischer und pathologischer Strukturen der Mamma unter Anwendung eines Immersionsscanners. Dissertation, University of Marburg, West Germany, pp. 15-43.

Ezo, MG. (1981). Tissue compression for the optimization of images in waterpath breast scanning. *Medical Ultrasound 5*:113-117.

Friedrich, M. (1981). Neue technische Entwicklungen der Röntgen- und Ultraschalluntersuchung der Mamma. *Röntgenpraxis 34*:181-195.

Friedrich, M., Claussen, C.C., Felix, R. (1981). Methodische Aspekte der Mammasonographie. Erfahrungen mit einem Immersionsscanner (Octoson). *RöFo 135*:704-713.

Gros, Ch.M., Dale, G., Gairard, B. (1978). La compression en échographie mammaire. *Senologia 3*:3-13.

Hackelöer, B.J., Duda, V., Hüneke, B., Lauth, G., Bald, R., Buchholz, R. (1982). Ultraschallmammographie: Entwicklung, Stand und Grenzen. *Ultraschall in der Medizin 3*:94-108.

Huber, J.C., Fischl, F., Kubista, E., Reinold, E. (1982). Real-time-Sonographie in der Mammaroutinediagnostik. *Ultraschall in der Medizin 3*:137-139.

Hüppe, J.R. (1982). Zur Technik der Mammasonographie mit Real-Time-Gerät. Lecture, Breast Sonography Conference, Munich, Sept. 24, Klinikum Grosshadern.

Kossoff, G. (1978). *Automated Ultrasonic Scanning Techniques*. Excerpta Medica, Amsterdam, pp. 22-35.

Kossoff, G., Jellins, J. (1982). The physics of breast echography. *Seminars in Ultrasound 3*:5-12.

Lauth, G., Duda, V., Hackelöer, B.J. (1984). Möglichkeiten und Grenzen der Interpretation von Ultraschall-Mammogrammen. *Röntgen-Berichte 13*:21-34.

Maturo, V.G., Zusmer, N.R., Gilson, A.J., Smoak, W.M., Janowitz, W.R., Bear, B.E., Goddard, J., Dick, D.E. (1980). Ultrasound of the whole breast utilizing a dedicated automated breast scanner. *Radiology 137*:457-463.

Picker, R.H., Fulton, A.J. (1982). Maturational and physiological changes in the female breast. *Seminars in Ultrasound 3*:34-37.

Rosensweig, R., Foy, P.M., Cole-Beuglet, C., Kurtz, A.B., Goldberg, B.B. (1982). Radial scanning of the breast: An alternative to the standard ultrasound technique. *Journal of Clinical Ultrasound 10*:199-201.

Sanders, R.C. (1980). Comparison between black and white backgrounds for ultrasonic images. *Journal of Clinical Ultrasound 8*:413-415.

Schneck, C.D., Lehmann, D.A. (1982). Sonographic anatomy of the breast. *Seminars in Ultrasound 3*:13-33.

Teubner, J., Müller, A., Pickenhan, I., van Kaick, G. (1982). Morphologie der Brustdrüse im Schallbild. In Kratochwil, Reinold (Eds.), *Ultraschalldiagnostik '81*. Thieme, Stuttgart, France, pp. 369-370.

Teubner, J., Müller, V., van Kaick, G. (1983). Echomorphologie der Brustdrüse. *Radiologe 23*:97-107.

Teubner, J., van Kaick, G., Pickenham, L., Schmidt, W. (1982). Vergleichende Untersuchung mit verschiedenen echomammographischen Verfahren. *Ultraschall in der Medizin 3*:109-118.

Van Kaick, G., Schmidt, W., Teubner, J., Lorenz, D., Lorenz, A., Müller, A. (1980). Echomammographie mit verschiedenen Gerätetypen bei herdförmigen Läsionen. *Tumordiagnostik 4*:179-186.

2
Benign Diseases

Duct Ectasia

Both normal and ectatic milk ducts are readily detected on breast sonograms (Fig. 2.1). Intraductal masses, however, cannot be reliably identified with ultrasound. As Fig. 2.2 illustrates, intraductal papillomas or carcinomas may produce internal echoes in dilated ducts, but these echoes are indistinguishable from the echoes that occur when the beam cuts normal duct walls tangentially. Thus, the presence of duct ectasia or a prominent ductal pattern on the sonogram of the nonlactating

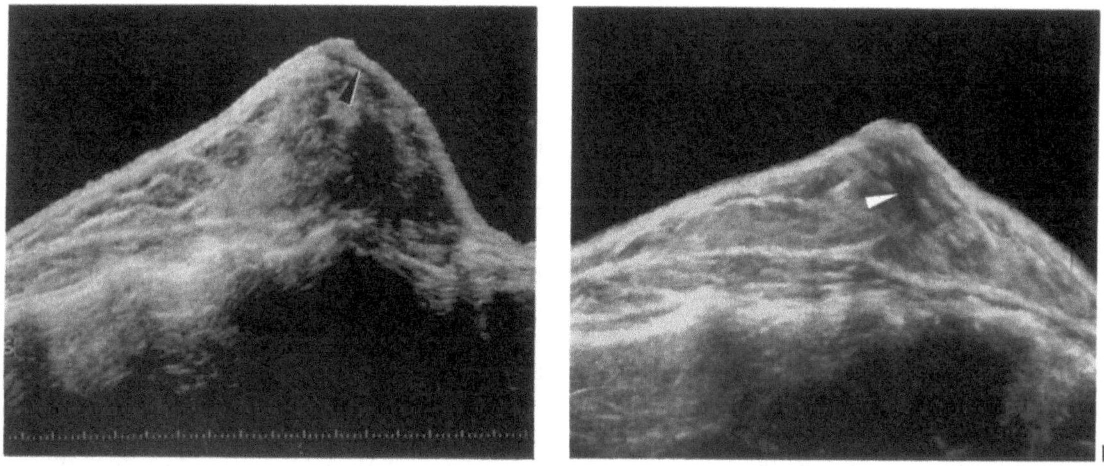

a b

Fig. 2.1. Sonogram of **a** undilated lactiferous duct, **b** duct ectasia

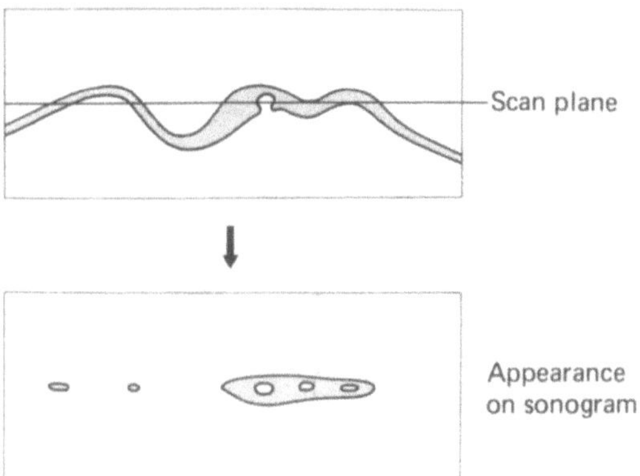

Fig. 2.2. "Intraductal" structures on sonogram

breast is an indication for further diagnostic evaluation by contrast ductography (see Chap. 5). It should be noted that large areas manifesting a ductal structure are less suspicious for disease than small, very prominent areas or isolated ectatic ducts.

Simple Cysts

Simple breast cysts (Fig. 2.3) are characterized sonographically by their echo-free (anechoic) interiors and smooth margins. While the anterior and especially the posterior margins are always sharply defined, the lateral boundaries may be indistinct as a result of reflective and refractive edge shadowing. Posterior acoustic enhancement is more or less pronounced owing to the anechoicity of the mass. The strength of this effect depends not only on the diameter of the cyst but also on its depth and the echogenicity of surrounding tissues. Because these factors are mutually independent, the degree of posterior enhancement in cysts is highly variable; one is just as likely to find relatively small cysts with strong enhancement as large cysts with weak enhancement. The better the adjustment of focusing and TGC the more perpendicular the beam incidence, and the more central the transit of the beam through the lesion the easier it is to appreciate the smooth margins, echo-free interior, and conspicuous secondary phenomena that are the hallmarks of uncomplicated breast cysts (Figs. 1.22, 2.4). Peripheral areas of the cyst can appear to have ill-defined margins and a solid internal structure, and these can mask secondary phenomena (Fig. 2.5). This often creates problems of differential diagnosis, especially with relatively small cysts. Confusion can also result from the projection of scattered echoes into the cysts from surrounding tissues. In doubtful cases, needle aspiration should be performed to clarify the nature of the lesion.

Uncomplicated breast cysts do not always occur as solitary round or oval masses; frequently they are multiple and lobulated and show interior lobulation or septation (Figs. 2.6–2.8). The ability to demonstrate intracystic septa or lobulated cysts with ultrasound is an important advantage, for it aids in the planning of needle aspirations and makes it easier to evacuate all compartments when the aspiration is carried out.

The role of sonography in the aspiration of cysts is discussed in more detail in the section on sonographic guidance of needle aspirations and biopsies in Chapter 5. Here we shall note only that every cyst that is to be aspirated should first be scrutinized with ultrasound to assess its margins and echogenicity. Afterward the aspirating needle is passed into the cyst under direct sonographic guidance, and the cyst is evacuated. A successful aspiration is signified by the complete disappearance of the mass on the monitoring screen. If residual fluid is noted, an attempt is made to remove it by adjusting the needle placement, repositioning the patient, or compressing the breast. After air has been injected to inhibit cyst refilling and prepare for pneumocystography, it is no longer possible to evaluate the aspirated cyst with ultrasound. The air produces a bright band along the former anterior cyst wall, with associated posterior shadowing. Occasionally an air crescent of this type will produce a "rope-ladder" pattern caused by multiple reverberations (Figs. 2.9–2.11).

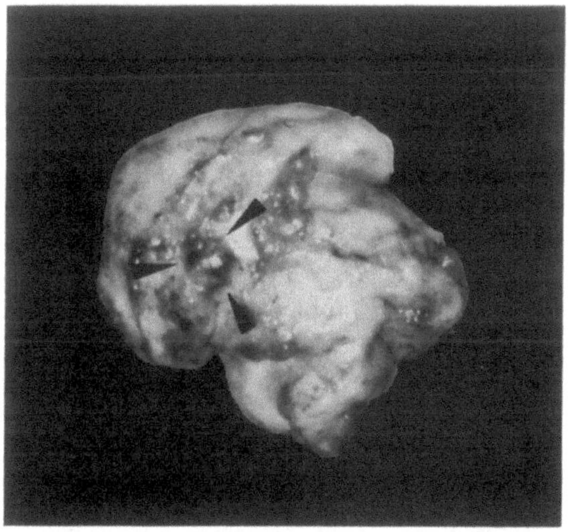

Fig. 2.3. Gross appearance of a simple breast cyst

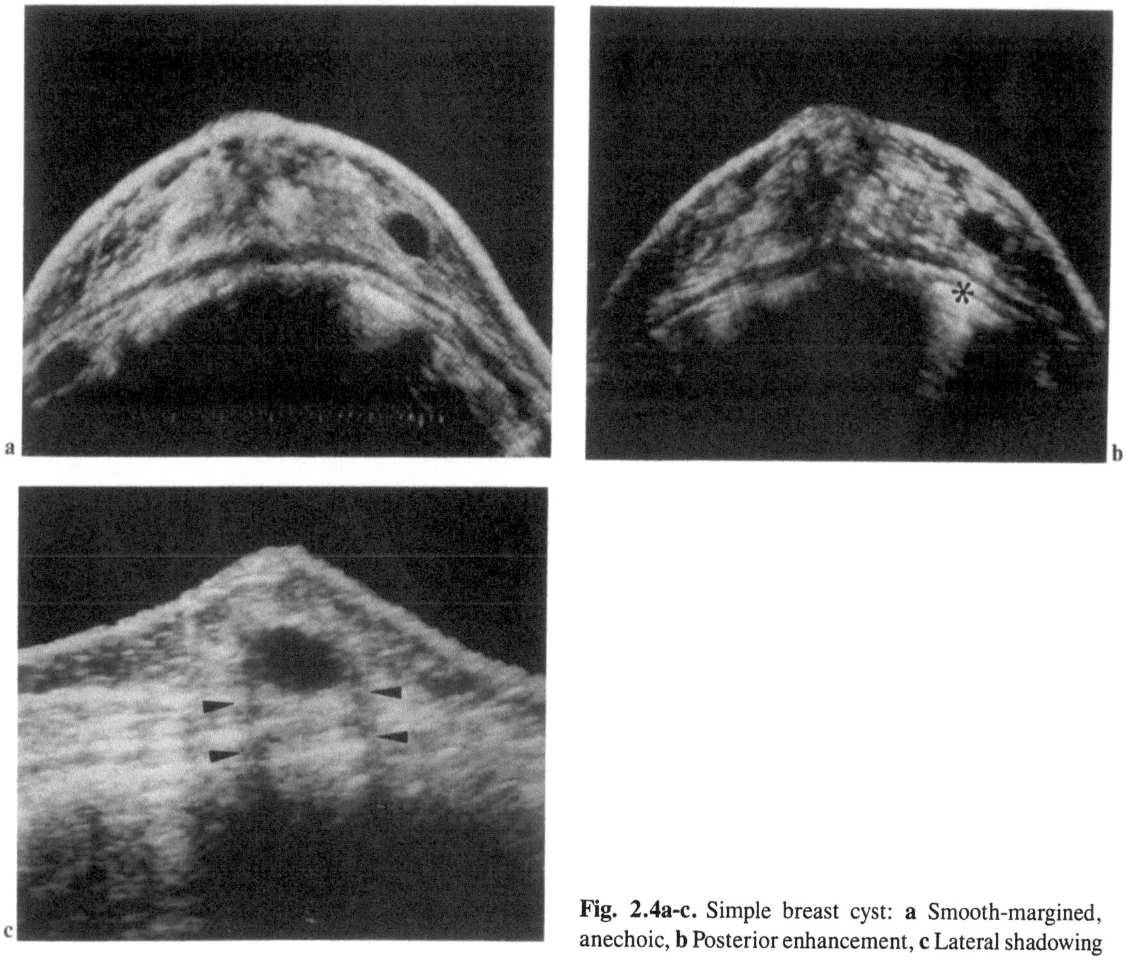

Fig. 2.4a-c. Simple breast cyst: **a** Smooth-margined, anechoic, **b** Posterior enhancement, **c** Lateral shadowing

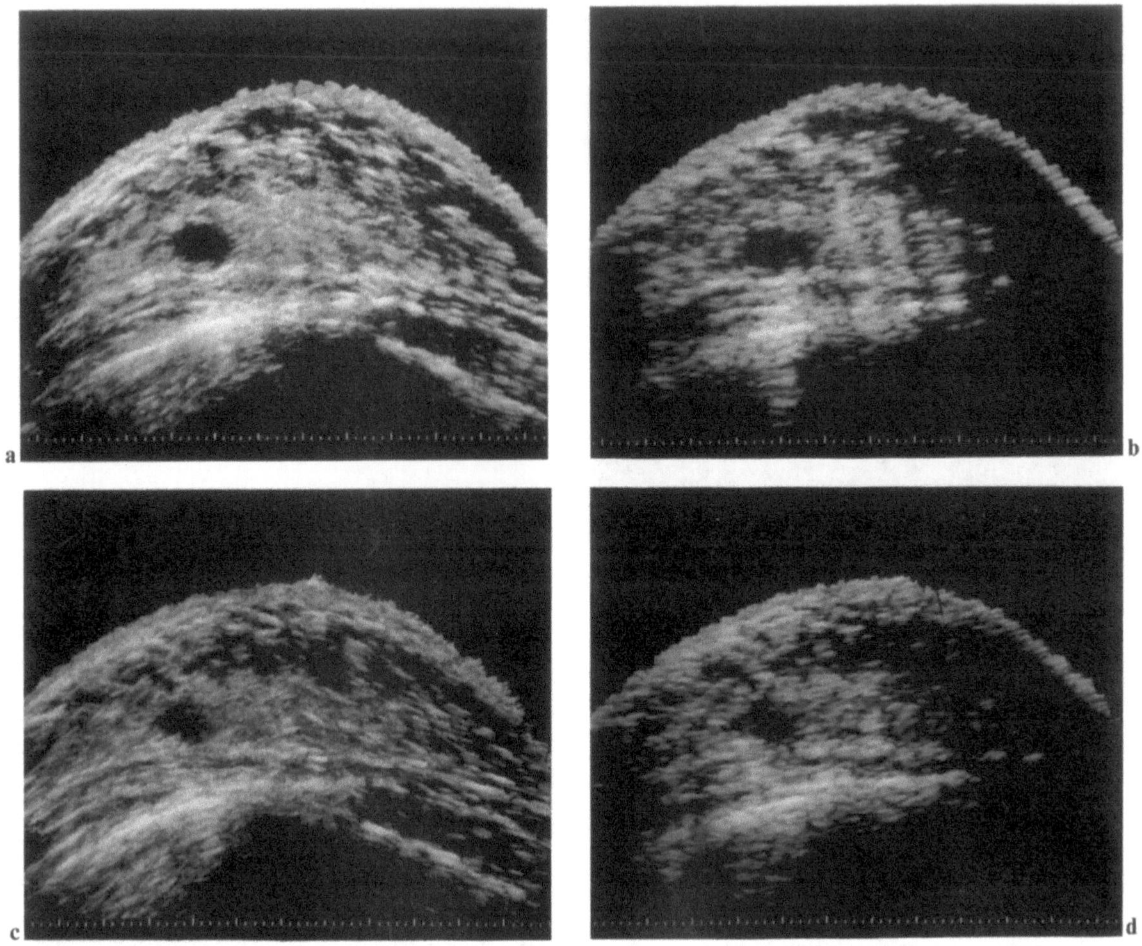

Fig. 2.5a,b. Scan traversing center of cyst (smooth-margined, anechoic, posterior enhancement). **c,d** Scan traversing periphery of cyst (poorly marginated, faint, no secondary phenomena)

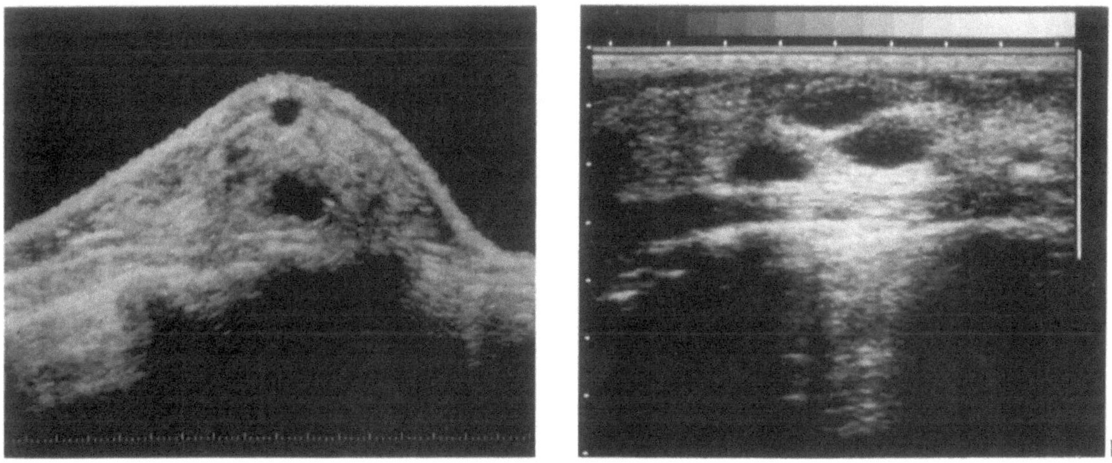

a b

Fig. 2.6a,b. Multiple cysts

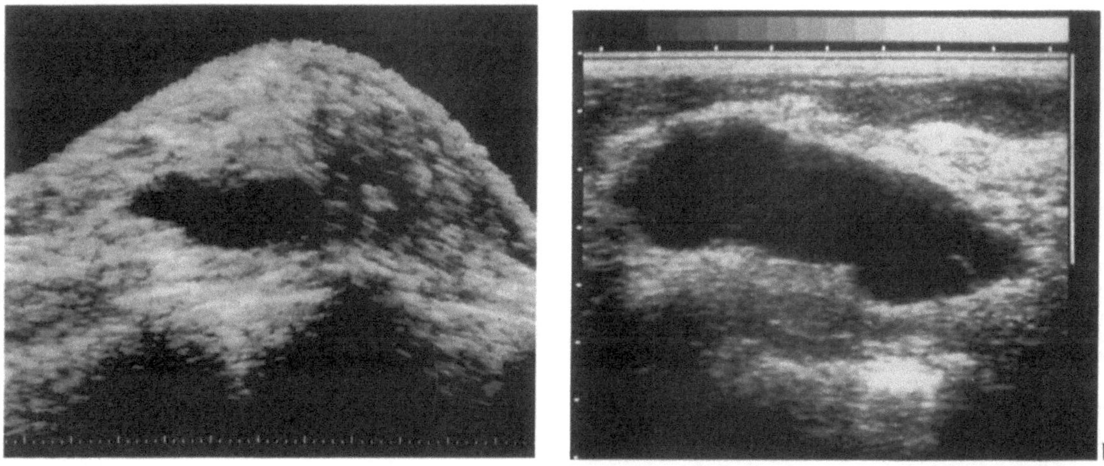

a b

Fig. 2.7a,b. Cysts with lobulated borders

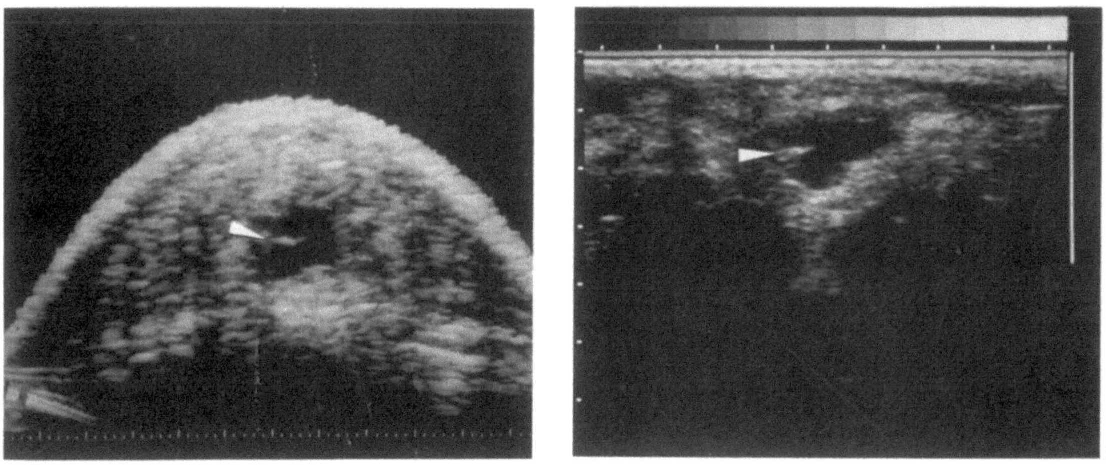

a b

Fig. 2.8a,b. Intracystic septa

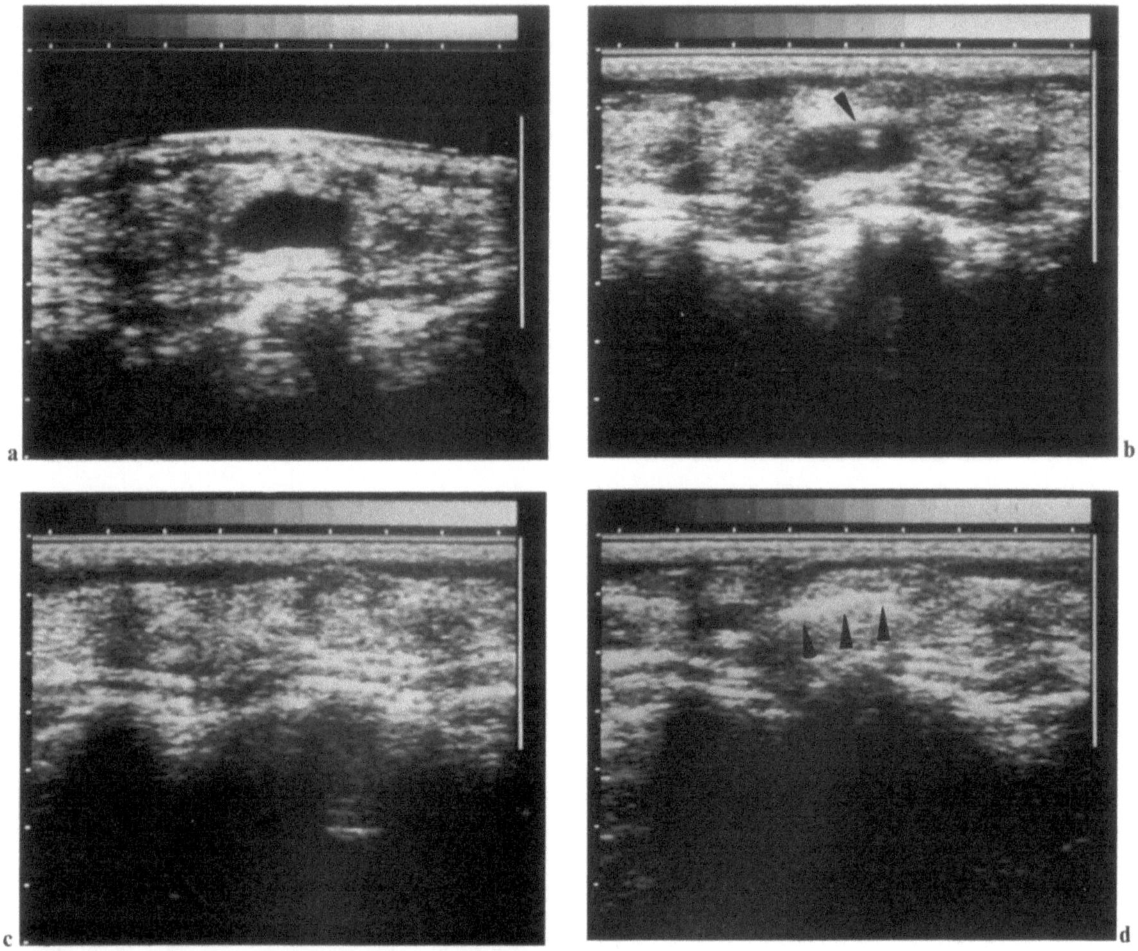

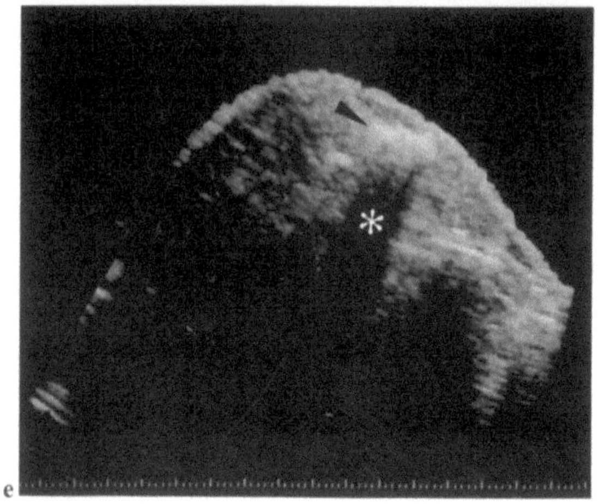

Fig. 2.9. **a** Cyst prior to aspiration (scan taken with coupling path). **b** Bright needle tip is visible within the cyst. **c** Postaspiration scan. **d**,**e** Hyperechoic crescents after air injection

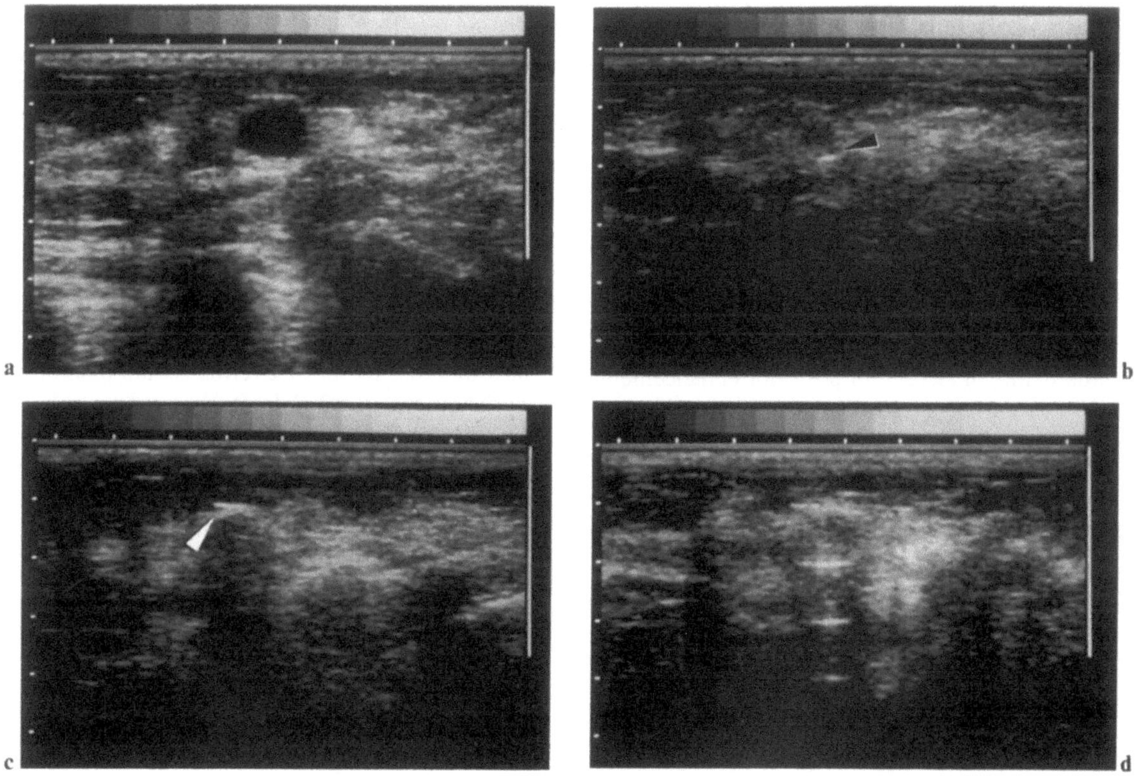

Fig. 2.10. **a** Cyst prior to aspiration. **b** Tip of needle following aspiration. **c** Air crescent. **d** "Rope-ladder" reverberations from the air crescent

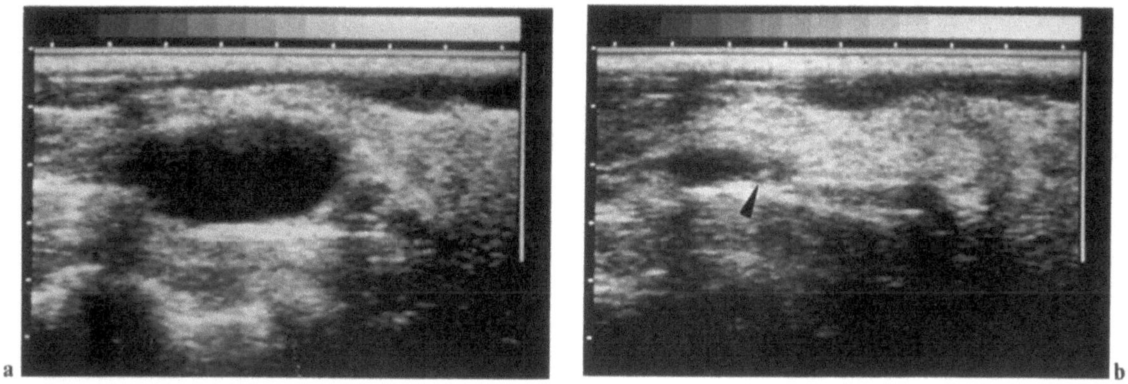

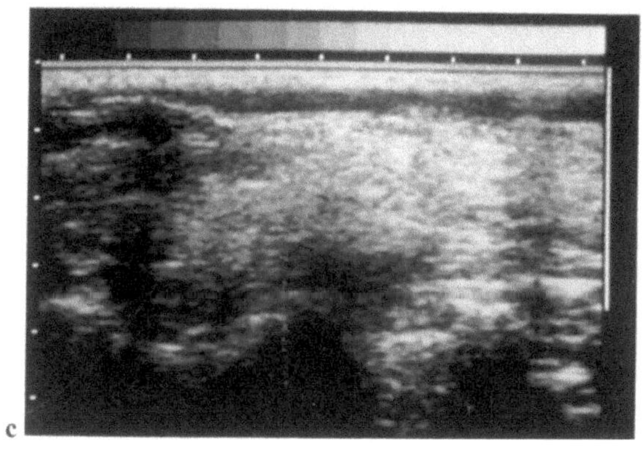

Fig. 2.11. **a** Cyst prior to aspiration. **b** Needle tip in partially evacuated cyst. **c** Complete evacuation.

Cysts with Internal Echoes

These lesions include primarily cystic masses with solid components as well as solid-appearing masses that show an association with cysts on further investigation. Because cystic-solid lesions of the breast can have numerous etiologies, this type of pattern calls for a very careful and precise diagnostic evaluation (Table 2.1, Fig. 2.12).

Sonograms may show either atypical-appearing cysts or solid masses that resemble cysts by virtue of their smooth margins or posterior enhancement (Figs. 2.12–2.16). Major parts of the preoperative diagnostic workup in these cases, besides a careful ultrasound examination, are pneumocystography and cytologic evaluation of aspirated material. Positive results of either of these calls for excisional biopsy. A sonographic diagnosis of "artifactual internal echoes in a simple breast cyst" is justified only with a completely normal pneumocystogram and negative cytology (corresponding to Papanicolaou class I/II). Even so, the patient should return for a follow-up sonogram within about 3 months. If the cyst refills within a short time after evacuation (2–3 days), an event possibly accompanied by the reappearance of a palpable mass, the aspiration should be repeated to ensure that an intracystic carcinoma, for example, is not missed.

Table 2.1. Differential diagnosis of cysts with internal echoes.

Artifactual internal echoes	Echoes scattered from surrounding tissues
	Scan through periphery of cyst (Fig. 2.5)
	Scan through wall of irregularly shaped cyst (Fig. 2.10)
True internal echoes	Incomplete cyst evacuation (Fig. 2.11)
	Special cystic contents (e.g., pasty, putrid, hemorrhagic; Fig. 2.12)
	Epidermoid cysts
	Intracystic papilloma (Fig. 2.13)
	Intracystic carcinoma (Fig. 2.14)
Other	Hematoma (Fig. 4.1–4.3)
	Abscess (Figs. 2.15–2.20)
	Bleeding within a solid mass (Fig. (3.20)
	Solid mass with special growth (e.g., mucinous or medullary carcinoma (Figs. 3.22–3.32)
	Partially necrotic tumor (Fig. 3.19)

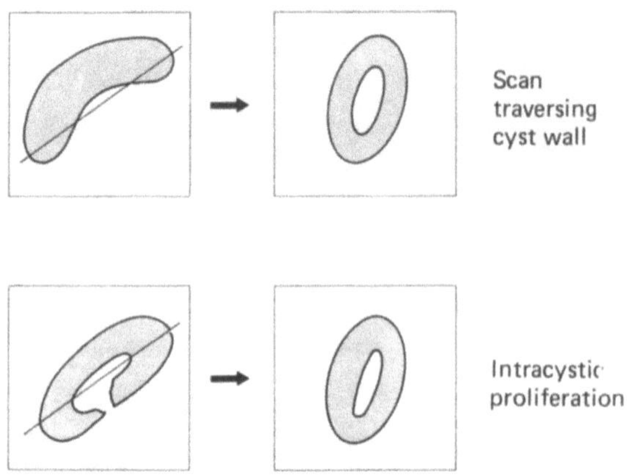

Fig. 2.12. Artificial and real causes for cysts "with internal echoes"

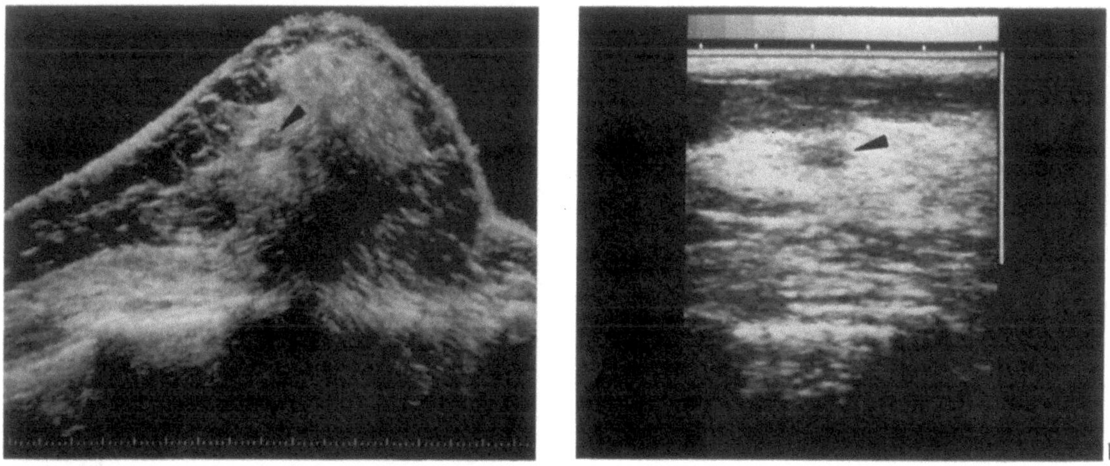

Fig. 2.13a,b. Appearance of breast on immersion scan (left) and real-time scan (right) 5½ weeks after incomplete cyst aspiration

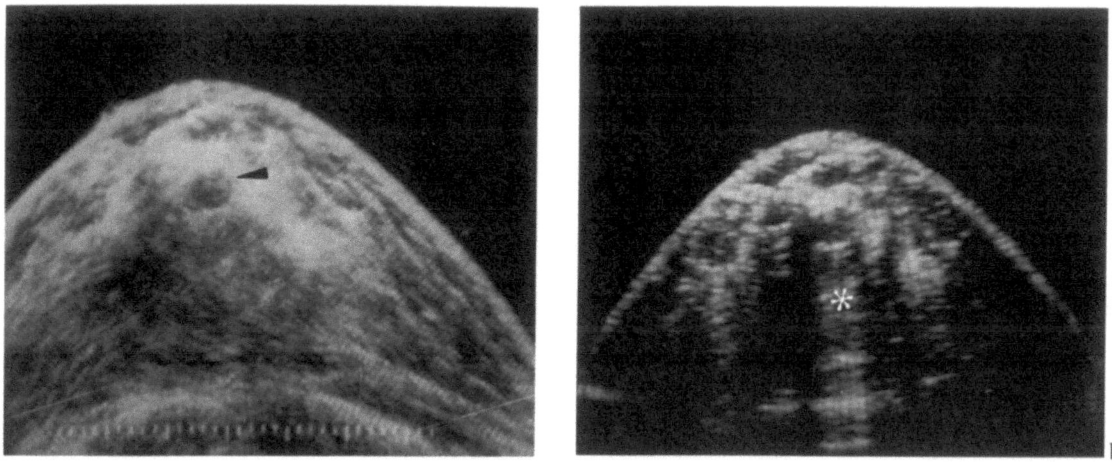

Fig. 2.14a,b. Cyst with pasty contents, appearing as a small "solid" mass with posterior enhancement

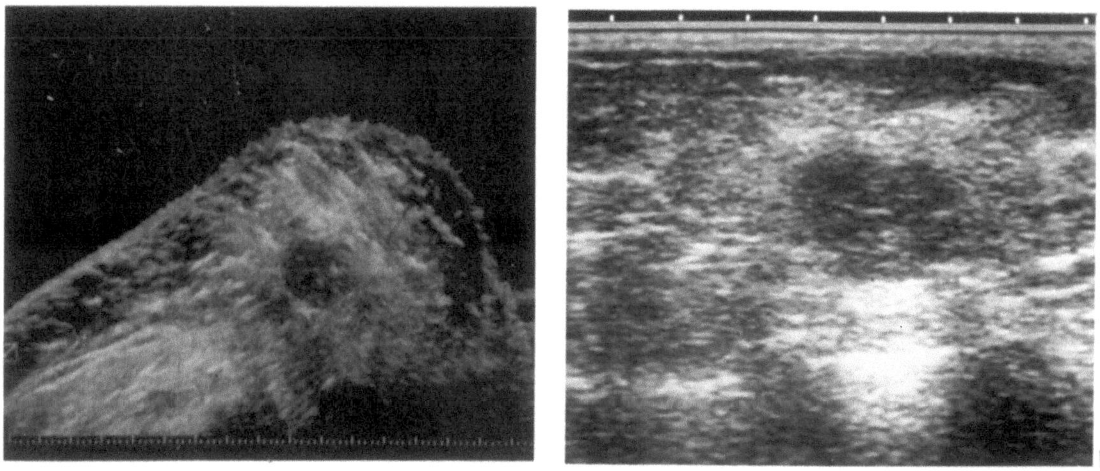

Fig. 2.15a,b. Intracystic papilloma: A firm 2.5-cm mass located at 2:00/8 cm in the left breast of a 69-year-old patient

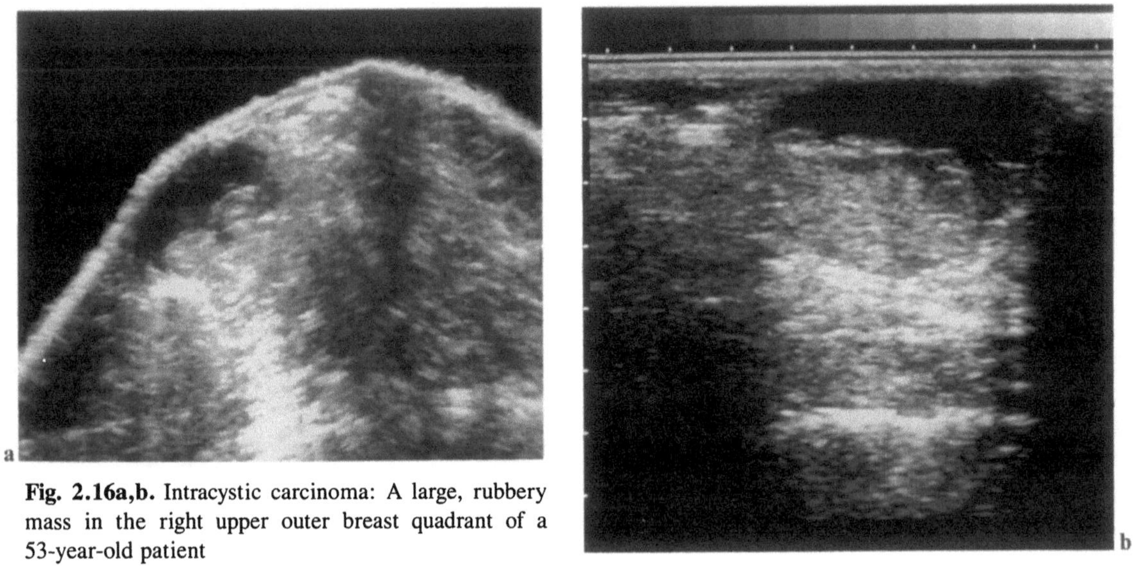

Fig. 2.16a,b. Intracystic carcinoma: A large, rubbery mass in the right upper outer breast quadrant of a 53-year-old patient

Mastitis

The mastitides can be grossly differentiated into puerperal, nonpuerperal, and granulomatous forms. The breast is also subject to other inflammatory disorders, such as folliculitis, that do not primarily involve the mammary gland (Table 2.2).

Inflammatory changes usually present sonographically as diverse or nonspecific structural alterations in the skin or glandular layer. Ultrasound in mastitis has major importance in the detection of abscesses, which present as anechoic or nearly anechoic areas with posterior enhancement (Figs. 2.19, 5.8). In many cases ultrasound can detect abscesses when they are still clinically occult. This can obviate the need for heat application to promote liquefaction and can shorten the overall duration of therapy.

Sonography is an ideal tool for monitoring the response of mastitis to antibiotic therapy (Fig. 2.20). It has only limited value in chronic mastitis with necrosis and cicatrization and in mastitic breasts that have been previously treated by incision (Fig. 2.21). Its value is similar limited by scars of other etiology (Figs. 4.3–4.5). Inflammatory carcinomas and mastitides are virtually indistinguishable on breast sonograms (Figs. 5.3, 5.4; Chap. 5).

Table 2.2. Different types of mastitis.

Type	Features
Puerperal mastitis	Main causal organisms: Staphylococci or streptococci Route of infection: Usually interstitial through infected nipple cracks, occasionally parenchymatous, i.e., hematogenous or ascending via the milk ducts as galactophoritis (Fig. 2.17)
Nonpuerperal mastitis	Infected cysts (aberrant milk ducts are common starting point in young women) (Fig. 2.18) Purulent mastitis with abscess formation (Fig. 2.19) Plasma cell mastitis (common around age 40 and in women with history of lactation problems) Nonspecific mastitis (often with necrosis and scarring) (Fig. 2.21)
Granulomatous mastitis	Foreign body granulomas Specific diseases (e.g., tuberculosis, Boeck's disease, leprosy, syphilis, actinomycosis, typhus) Mycoses (e.g., sporotrichosis, blastomycosis) Parasitic diseases (e.g., hydatid disease, cysticercosis, filariasis, schistosomiasis)
Folliculitis (Fig. 2.22)	

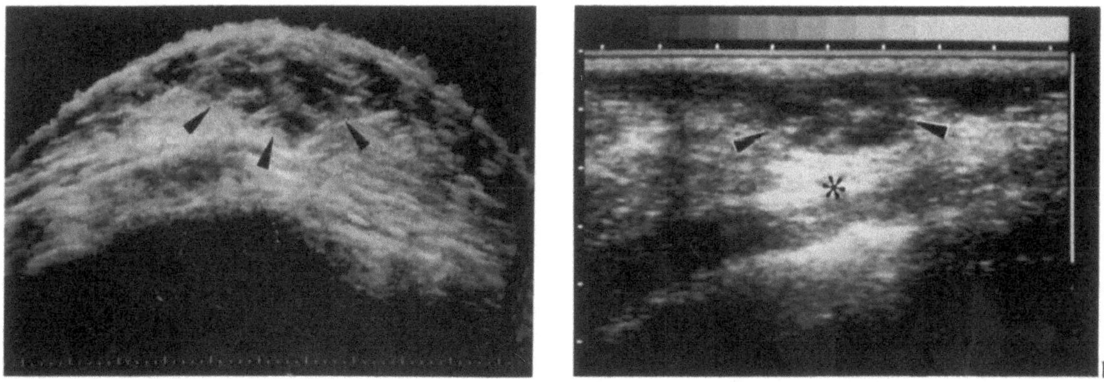

a b

Fig. 2.17a,b. Galactophoritis 8 days postpartum: An area of marked duct ectasia and enhancement occurs around a 2.5-cm, well-delineated, tender breast mass. On aspiration 3 ml of milky fluid was obtained

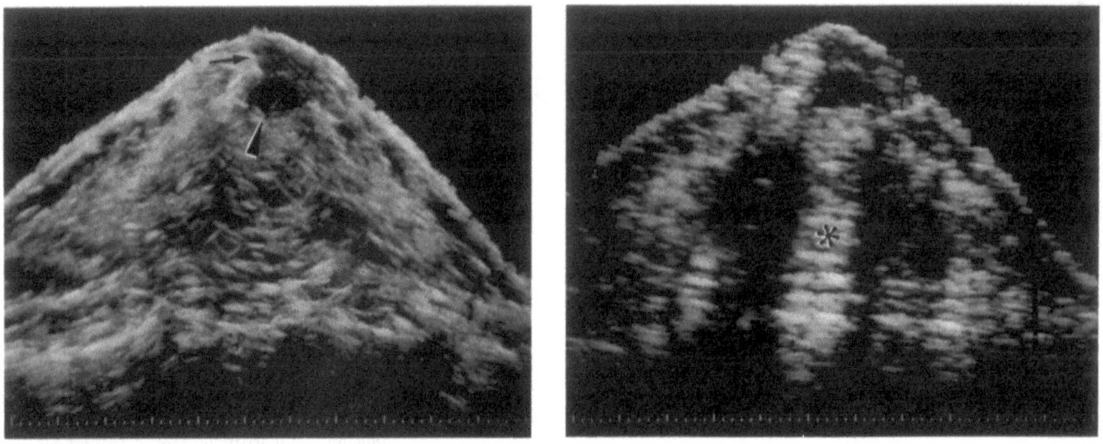

a b

Fig. 2.18a,b. Infected cyst in a 14-year-old girl. Sonogram shows hypoechoic mottling and expansion of the inflamed tissue above and around the cyst

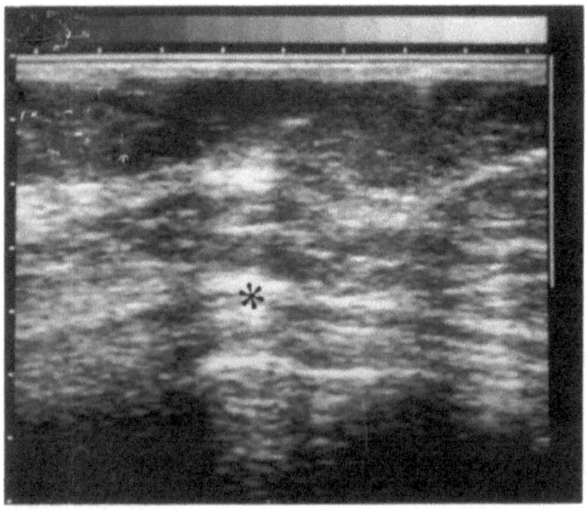

Fig. 2.19. Mastitis with abscess formation: Poorly marginated, nearly anechoic mass with marked posterior enhancement

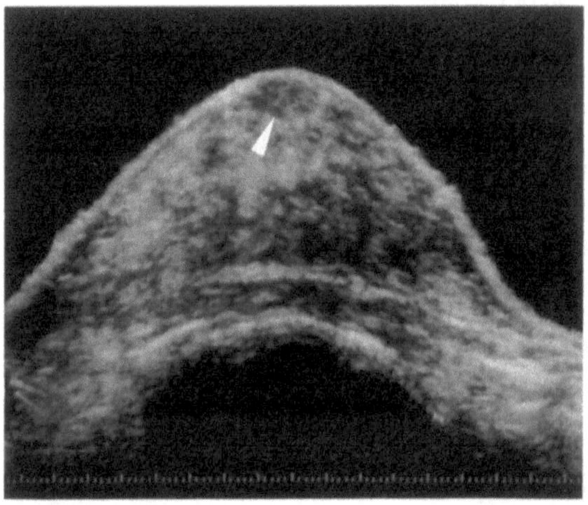

Fig. 2.20. Mastitis following antibiotic therapy: solid mass with no evidence of larger abscesses

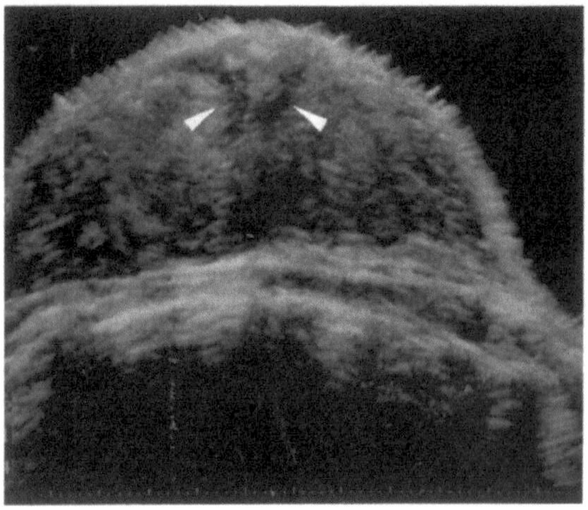

Fig. 2.21. Chronic mastitis with scars and calcifications.

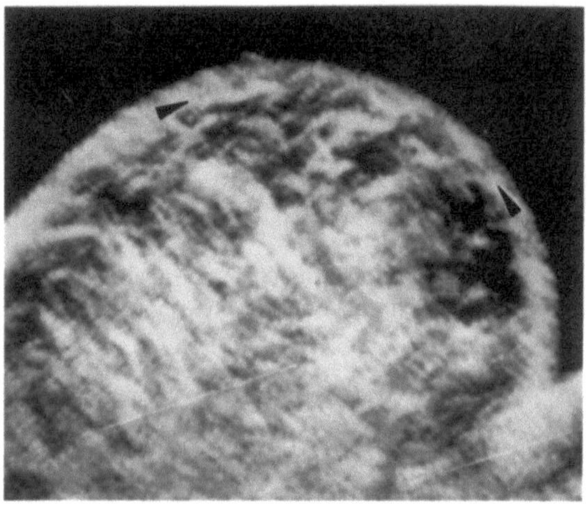

Fig. 2.22. Folliculitis with marked skin thickening

Rare Benign Breast Tumors

This group includes a variety of diseases that can produce tumorlike changes in the breast (Table 2.3). Understandably, the sonographic appearance of these changes is highly diverse, and they can be difficult to distinguish from malignancies. The examples that follow are intended more to illustrate the diagnostic problems that can arise than to facilitate identification.

Lipoma and Fat Necrosis

On X-ray mammograms, lipomas usually produce only an apparent absence of glandular parenchyma in the area of a palpable mass (Fig. 2.19a). On sonograms, lipomas present as more or less discrete masses whose echogenicity matches that of the rest of the fatty tissue, and which may show posterior enhancement (Fig. 2.23). Circumscribed lipomas may be indistinguishable from areas of involution into the glandular tissue.

Fat necrosis, like lipoma, is often detectable clinically as a palpable mass. Both sonographically and radiographically, the lesions of fat necrosis can often mimic carcinoma. Sonograms usually show a hypoechoic mass with ill-defined margins that may exhibit acoustic shadowing (Fig. 2.24). In approximately 200 women with fat necrosis, Bässler (1978) found a palpable mass in 100% and skin retraction in about 50% but noted a history of previous breast trauma in only about 40%. A correct clinical diagnosis was made in only 20% of patients, and a presumptive diagnosis of carcinoma was made in 28%. These results led Bässler to stress the "need for pathologic confirmation"—a position that is amply supported by previous experience with sonography.

Sonograms occasionally reveal small, round, well-defined anechoic foci in the subcutaneous fat layer. These areas, which yield a yellowish, fatty material when aspirated, can be most readily identified as oil cysts associated with fat necrosis and differentiated from true breast cysts on the basis of their localization (Fig. 2.25).

Granular Cell Tumors

These tumors usually present ill-defined margins and an irregular structure on sonograms, and many are indistinguishable from malignancies (Fig. 2.26). Their prevalence is very low: Only about 7% of all granular cell tumors occur in the breast (Bässler, 1978).

Table 2.3. Rare benign breast tumors.

Hemangiomas and lymphangiomas	Leiomyomas
Fibroepitheliomas	Lipomas
Fibromas	Granular cell tumors
Sclerodermatous tumors	Chondromas
Neurofibromas (Recklinghausen's disease)	Osteomas
	Adenomas
Histiocytomas	Adenomyotheliomas

Modified from Bässler, with permission.

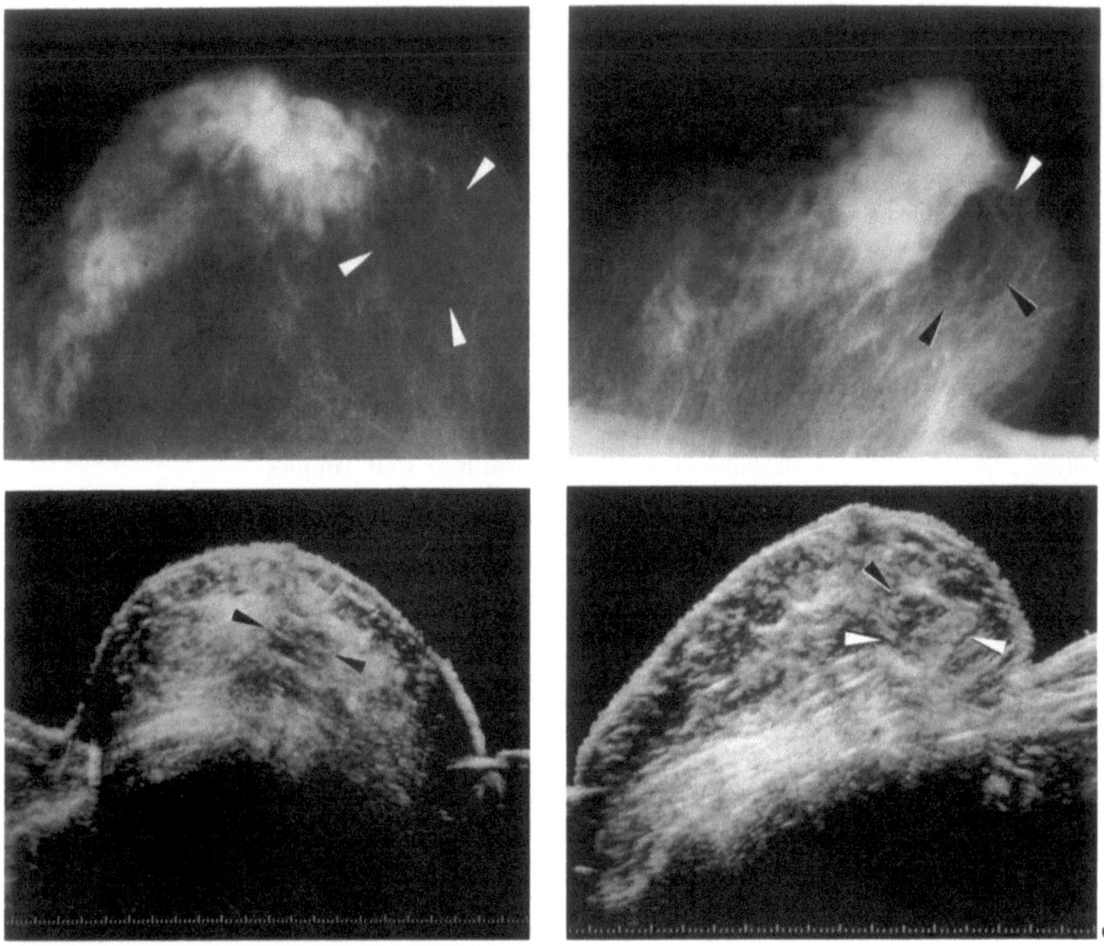

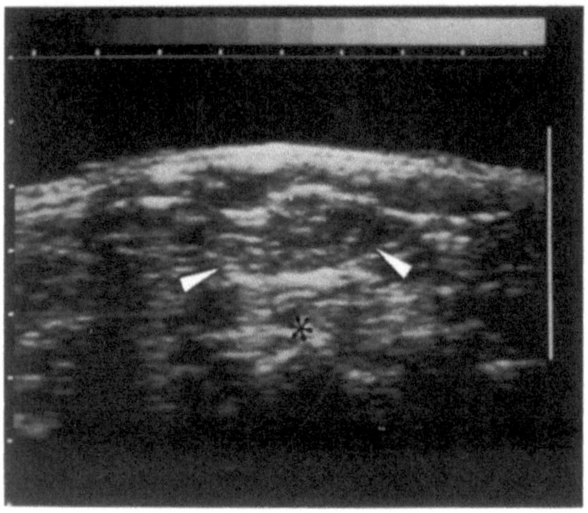

Fig. 2.23a-e. Lipoma. **a** X-ray mammograms, **b** immersion scans, and **c** real-time scan of 3×2-cm, well-demarcated, mobile tumor at 8:00/3 cm in the left breast of a 76-year-old woman

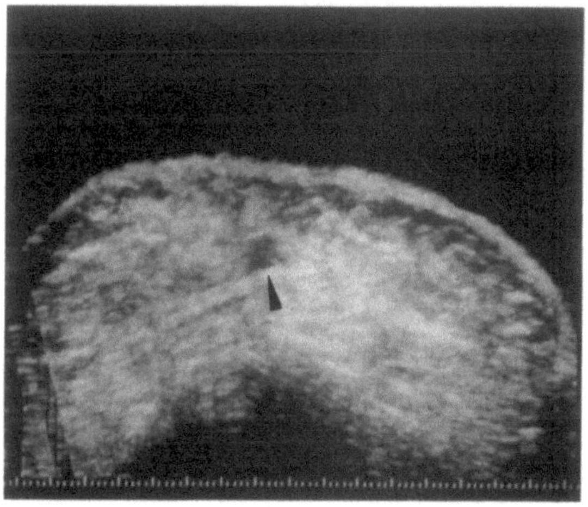

Fig. 2.24. Fat necrosis. A small, firm mass at 11:00/5.5 cm in the left breast of a 50-year-old woman following tumor excision 6 years previously

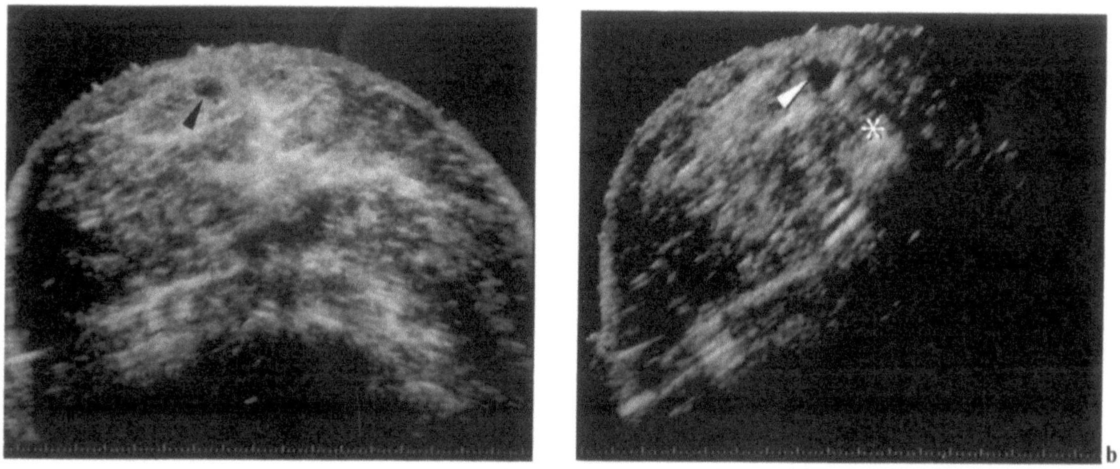

a b

Fig. 2.25a,b. Oil cysts. A small cystic mass in the subcutaneous fat layer about 14 days after blunt trauma. Aspiration yielded a fatty, oily fluid

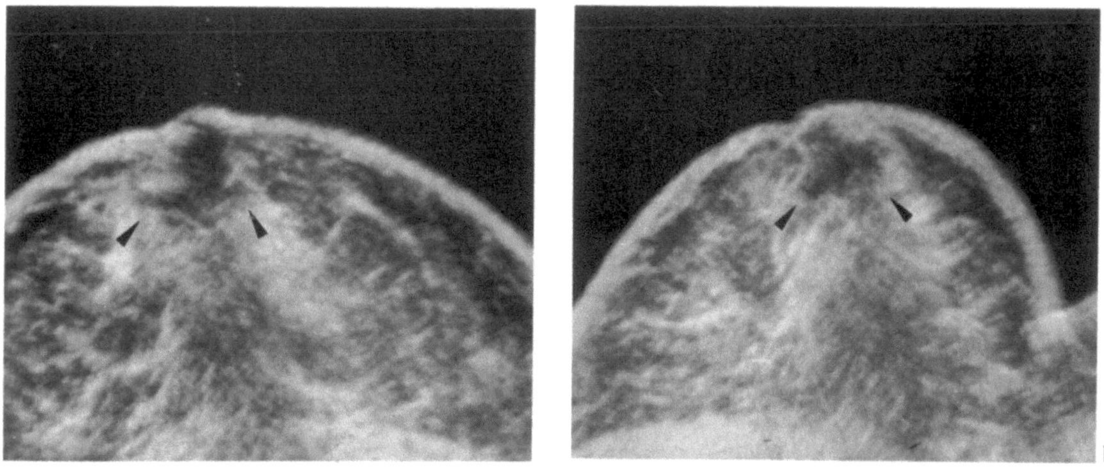

a b

Fig. 2.26a,b. Granular cell tumor. A firm 2-cm mass slightly above and lateral to the nipple in the right breast of a 69-year-old woman. The patient had a slightly positive Jackson sign and a brownish nipple discharge

Fibroadenomas

Fibroadenomas are the third most common type of breast lesion, surpassed in frequency only by carcinoma and fibrocystic disease. Fibroadenoma is the most common tumor in young women and typically occurs as a solitary, rounded, well-circumscribed mass 2 to 3 cm in size with a firm to rubbery consistency (Fig. 2.27). Bässler (1978) reported that the growth is multiple in 12.6% of cases (Fig. 2.31) and bilateral in only 4.2%. Sixty percent of fibroadenomas are 1 to 5 cm in diameter, and they rarely exceed 6 cm (Fig. 2.37). Most fibroadenomas grow relatively slowly, but occasionally they may show intense proliferation, especially during puberty, during pregnancy, and just before the menopause.

Fibroadenomas appear on sonograms as rounded masses with smooth margins and weak internal echoes. They are distinguishable from fibroadenosis and fibroadenomatoid hyperplasia by their surrounding capsule of displaced and compressed tissue, which creates a "halo" on the sonogram. This capsule, like smooth cyst walls, can produce lateral shadowing as a result of reflective and refractive processes. The internal echoes of fibroadenoma generally present a uniform distribution and regular structure. This fact bears on the observation that approximately one fourth of fibroadenomas depicted on sonograms show posterior acoustic enhancement. Table 2.4 shows the frequency of the various ultrasound criteria for fibroadenoma.

While the internal echoes of fibroadenomas present a "grainy" appearance on hand-held real-time scans, a "leafy" texture is more characteristic of immersion scans (Figs. 2.28–2.30). This "leafy" structure, which resembles fat, can occasionally make it difficult to distinguish peripherally situated fibroadenomas from the subcutaneous fat layer or involuted areas when the immersion technique is used. The hand-held real-time method with its compressive effect can be a helpful adjunct in these cases (Figs. 2.32, 2.33). Even with compression, fibroadenomatoid hyperplasia can be difficult to distinguish from other lesions due to the absence of a capsule or halo (Fig. 2.34).

Fibroadenomas that have an atypical sonographic appearance due to ill-defined margins or irregular, nonhomogeneous internal echoes may prove to be innocent on pathologic examination (Fig. 2.35), and others may show pathohistologic abnormalities (Fig. 2.36). Regarding the malignant transformation of fibroadenomas, Bässler (1978)

Table 2.4. Ultrasound criteria for fibroadenoma, according to frequency.

Criteria	Frequency (%)
Primary	
Margins	
Smooth	60
Halo	71
(Lateral shadowing	45)
Ill defined	12
Broom-straw pattern	0
Fir-tree pattern	0
Partially smooth	29
Internal echoes	
Uniform distribution	82
Regular structure	68
Non-uniform distribution	17
Irregular structure	12
Anechoic areas in the mass	0
Hyperechoic areas in the mass	30
Weak echo pattern	28
Secondary	
Posterior acoustic enhancement	
Behind portions of the mass	1
Behind the entire mass	24
Behind the entire mass on both planes	13
Acoustic shadowing	
Lateral	45
Central	5
Central on both planes	5

stated that “causal connections can exist between fibroadenoma and carcinoma or sarcoma in rare instances” and that “it is possible for fibroadenomas to harbor a malignant potential,” but he added that fibroadenoma “generally cannot be considered to be a precancerous or presarcomatous tumor.”

An unusually large mass whose sonographic features resemble fibroadenoma may well represent the rare case of a “giant fibroadenoma” that has reached a diameter of 6 cm or more (Fig. 2.37). But it may also represent the pathologically similar cystosarcoma phylloides, especially if the tumor is multilobular (Fig. 2.38). These tumors account for only 0.3% of all breast tumors and 2 to 3% of all fibroadenomas (Bässler, 1978).

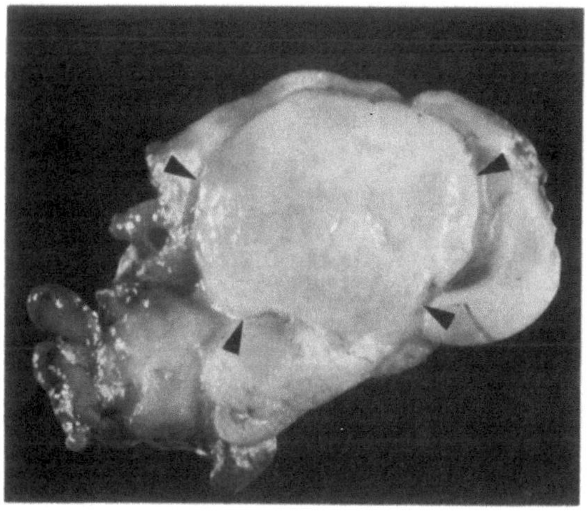

Fig. 2.27. Gross appearance of a fibroadenoma

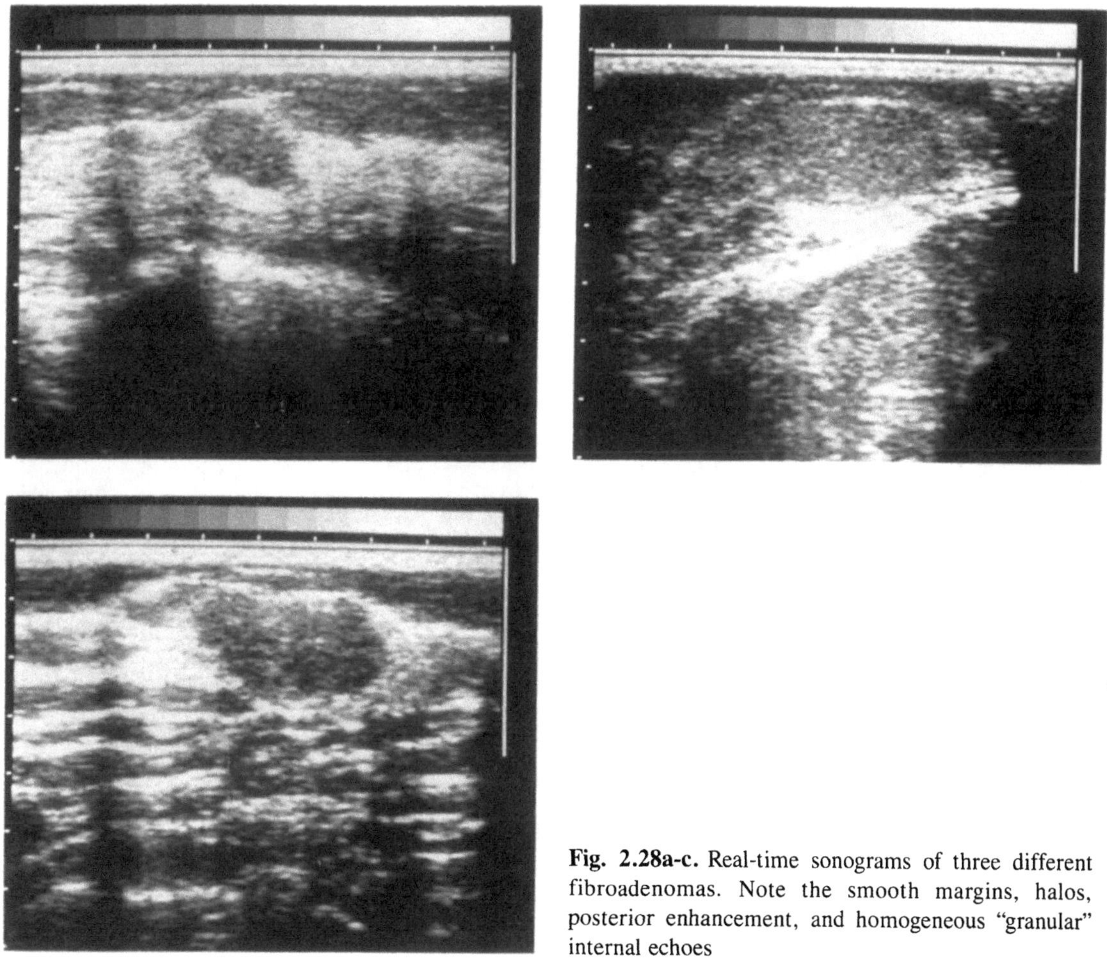

a b c

Fig. 2.28a-c. Real-time sonograms of three different fibroadenomas. Note the smooth margins, halos, posterior enhancement, and homogeneous “granular” internal echoes

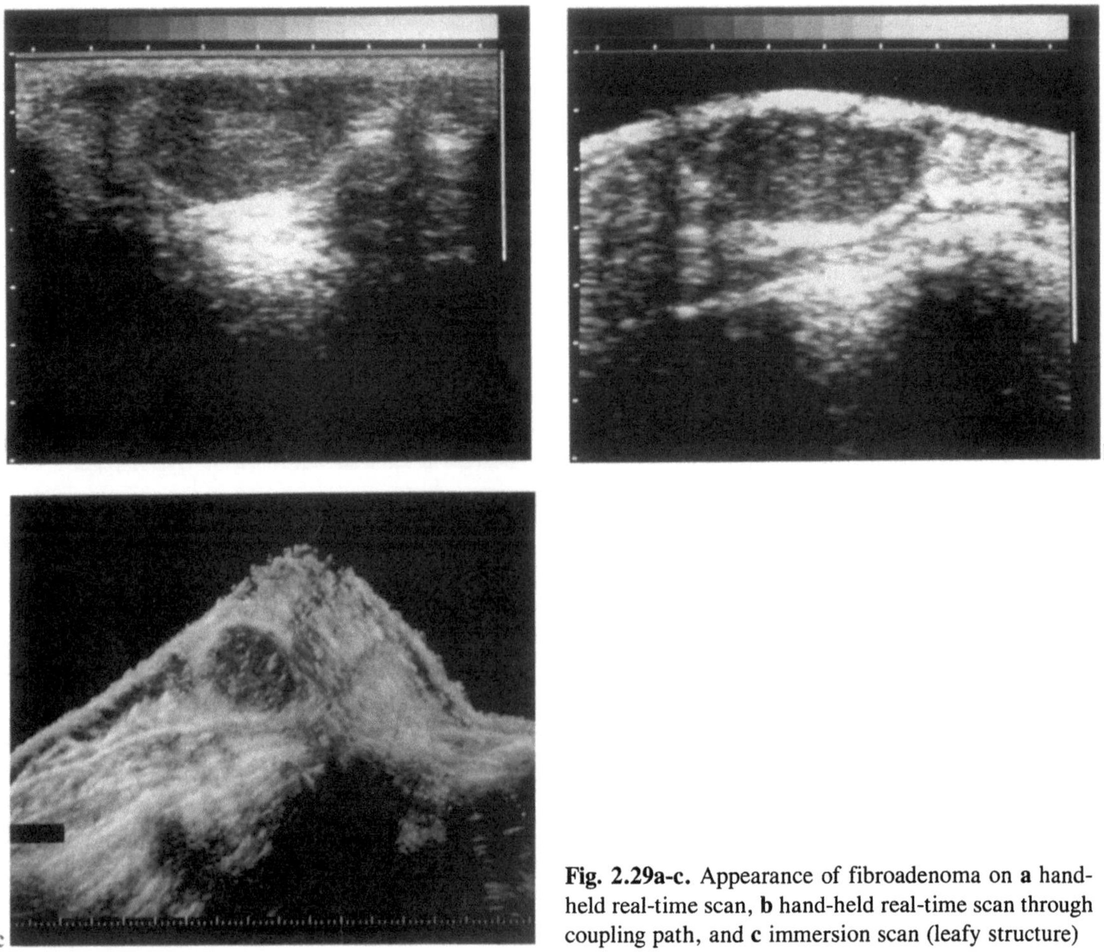

a b c

Fig. 2.29a-c. Appearance of fibroadenoma on a hand-held real-time scan, b hand-held real-time scan through coupling path, and c immersion scan (leafy structure)

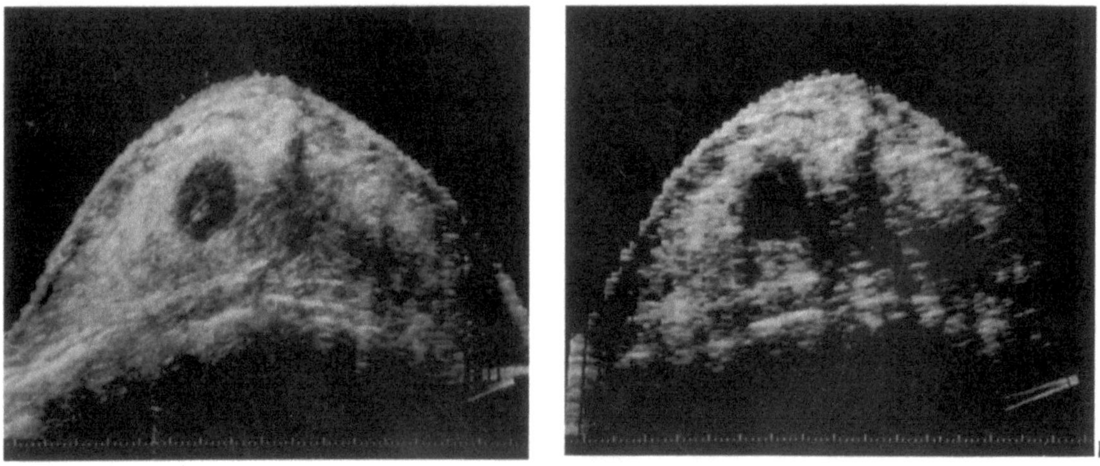

a b

Fig. 2.30a,b. Immersion scan of fibroadenoma with lateral shadowing

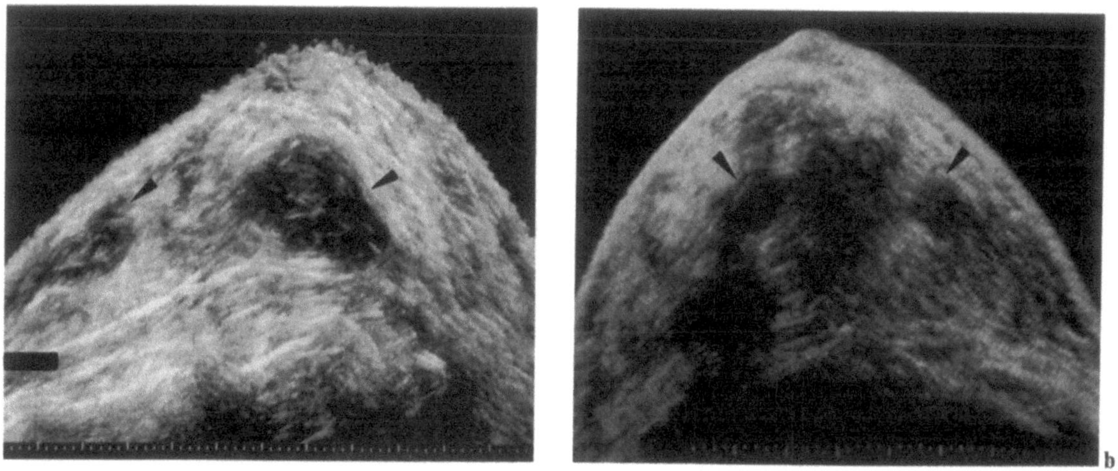

a b

Fig. 2.31a,b. Multiple fibroadenomas in (**a**) a 20-year-old woman and (**b**) a 22-year-old woman

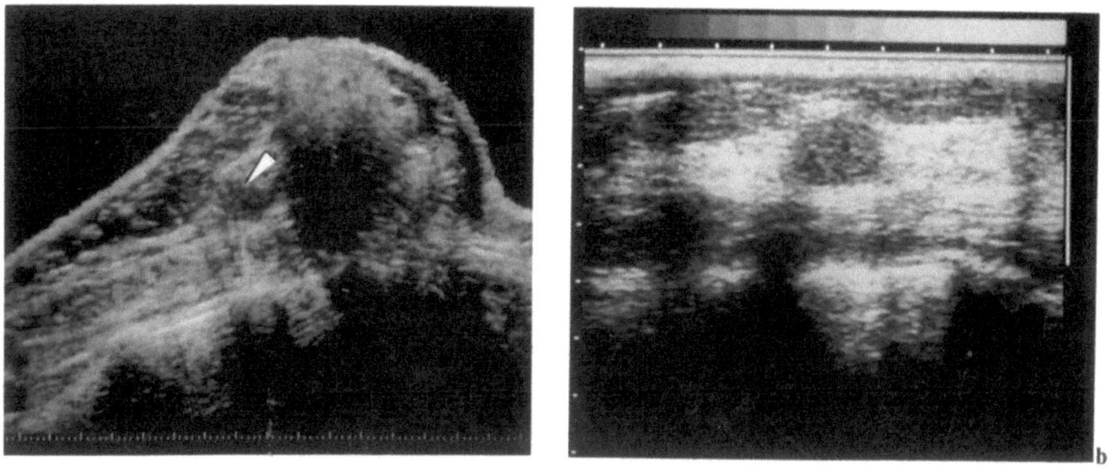

a b

Fig. 2.32a,b. Fibroadenoma measuring 1.8 cm in a 49-year-old woman. The mass is poorly delineated on the immersion scan (left) and well delineated on the real-time scan (right)

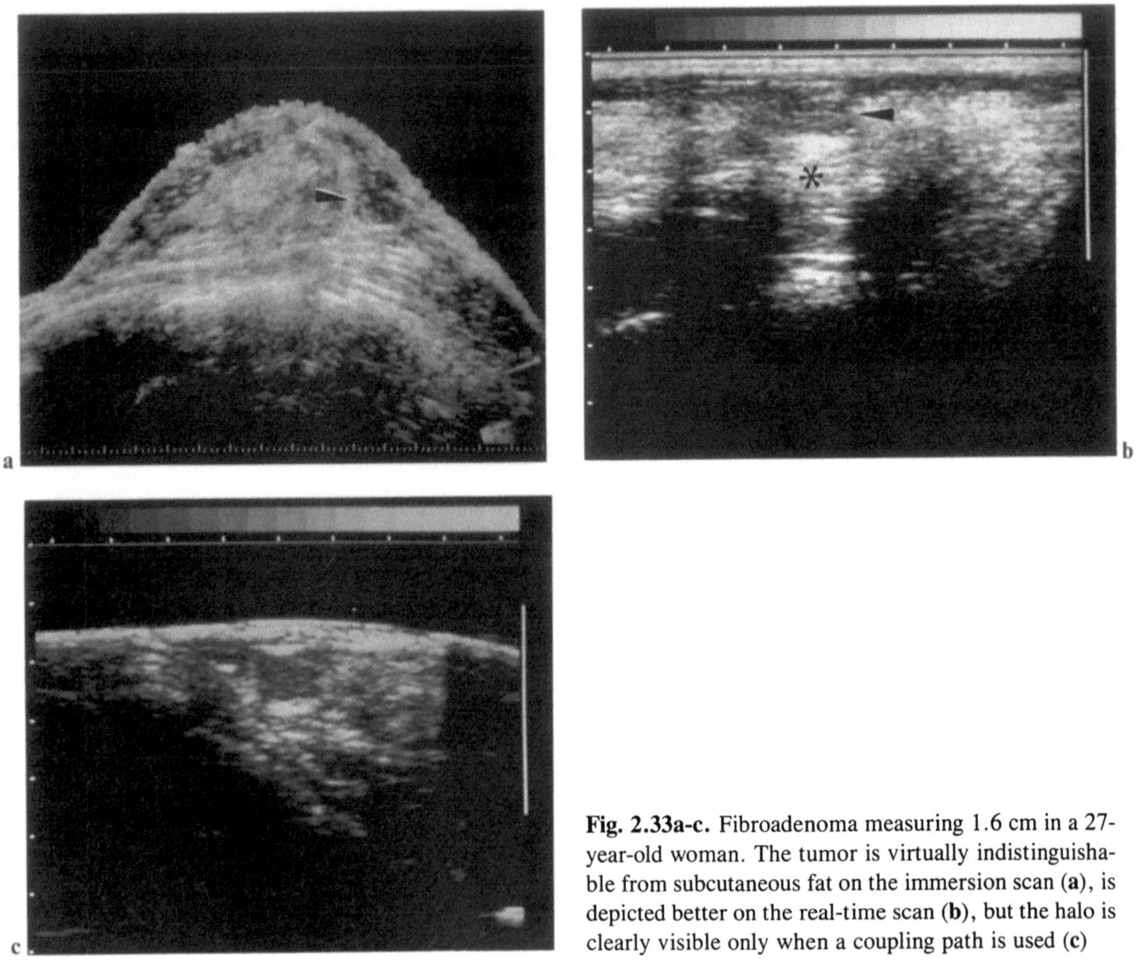

Fig. 2.33a-c. Fibroadenoma measuring 1.6 cm in a 27-year-old woman. The tumor is virtually indistinguishable from subcutaneous fat on the immersion scan (**a**), is depicted better on the real-time scan (**b**), but the halo is clearly visible only when a coupling path is used (**c**)

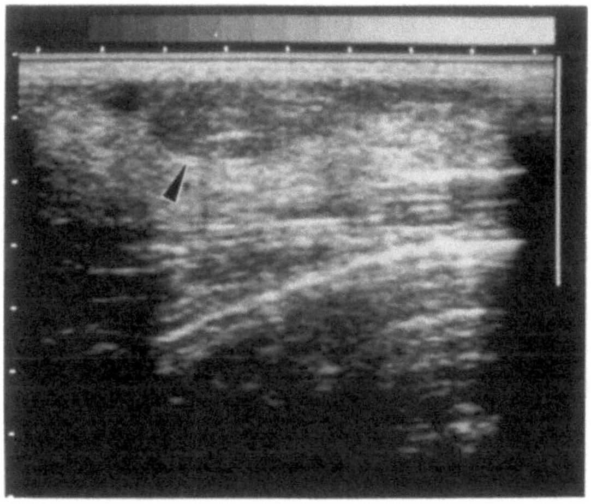

Fig. 2.34. Fibroadenomatoid hyperplasia: 4×3-cm mass at 2:00/2 cm in the left breast of a 24-year-old woman. Even with compression, the lesion is difficult to appreciate with ultrasound

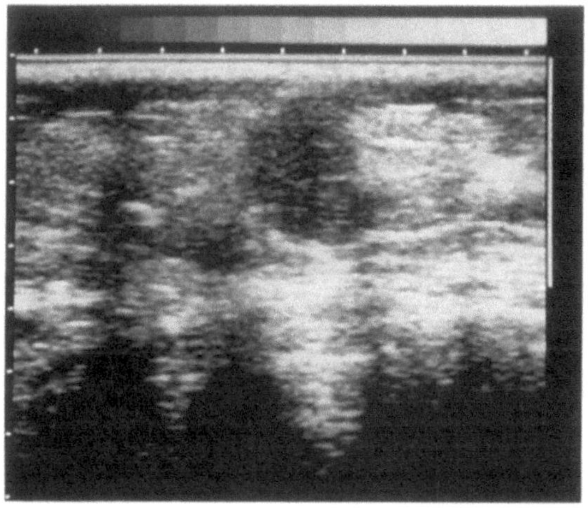

Fig. 2.35. Sonographically ill-defined 3×2-cm mobile breast mass in a 45-year-old woman. The lesion proved histologically to be an ordinary fibroadenoma

a 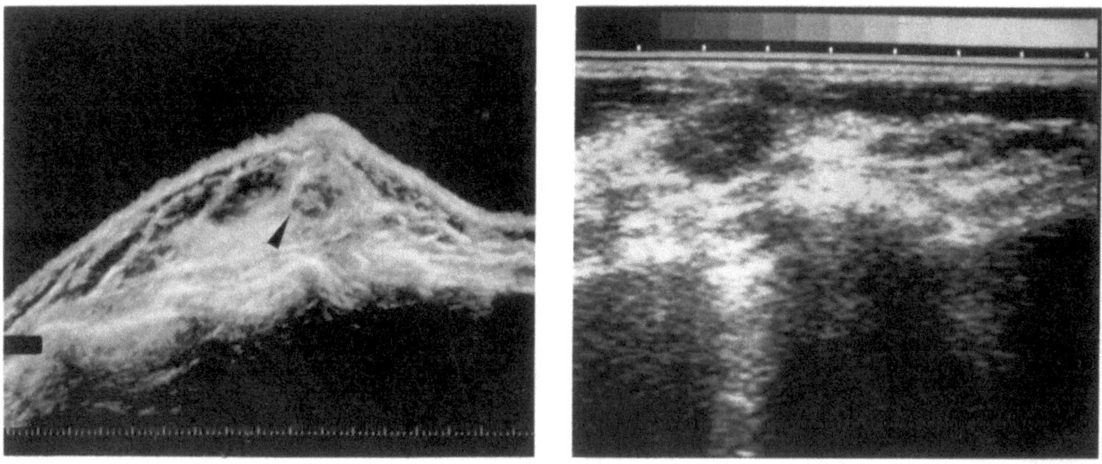 b

Fig. 2.36a,b. 1.5-cm fibroadenoma with cell atypia at 2:00/5 cm in the right breast of a 54-year-old woman

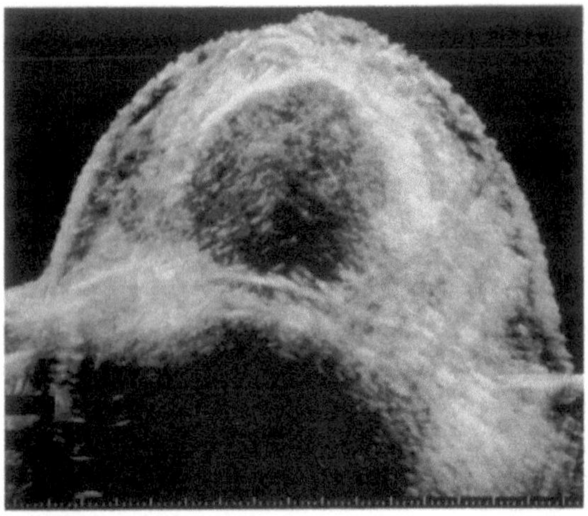
a

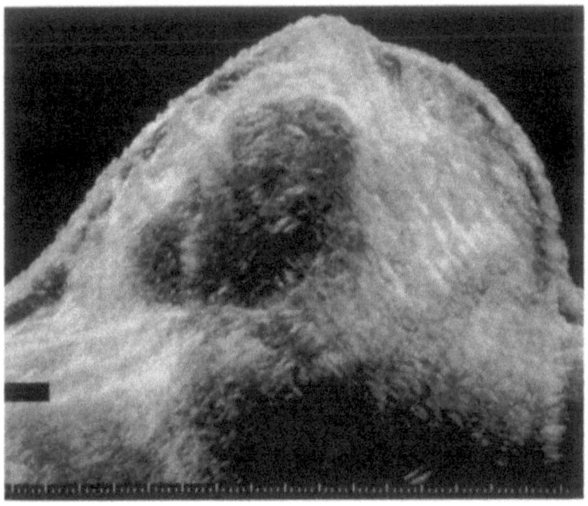
b

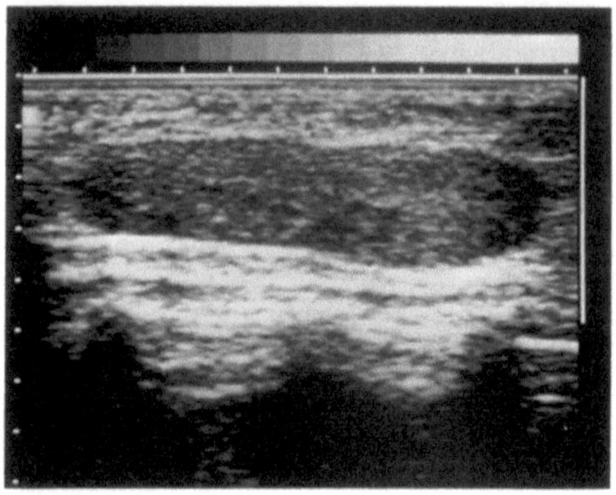
c

Fig. 2.37. Benign fibroadenoma measuring 10.5×6.2×2 cm in a 19-year-old woman. Note the marked compressibility of the mass

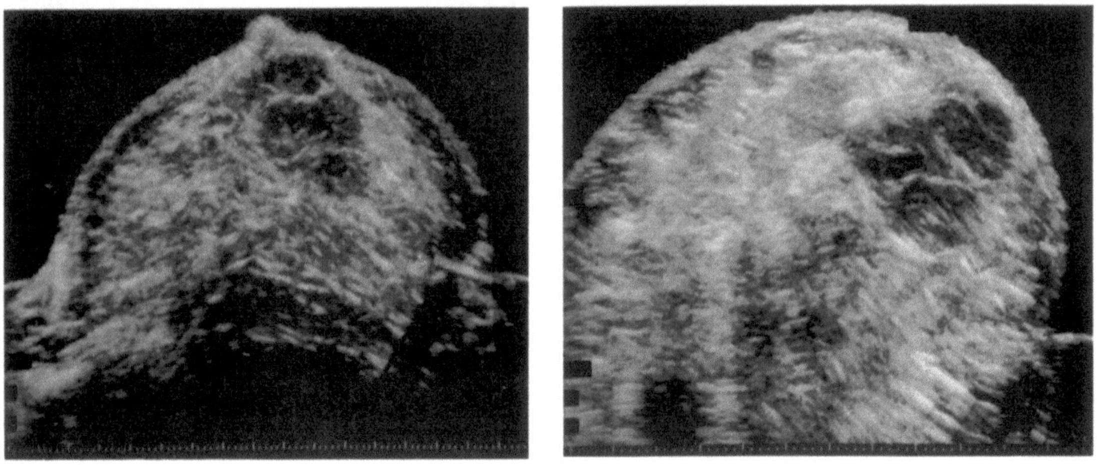
a b

Fig. 2.38a,b. Multilobular cystosarcoma phylloides in an 18-year-old woman

Diffuse Benign Breast Diseases

There are a number of diffuse, benign diseases of the breast that do not produce discrete, tumor-like changes. The main types are listed in Table 2.5.

Fibrocystic Disease

Fibrocystic disease ("mastopathy") is the most common diffuse breast disease. According to Bässler (1978), it occurs most commonly from 35 to 55 years of age, and thus before the menopause, and could be diagnosed in approximately 51% of 3000 unselected autopsies. Three grades of fibrocystic disease are recognized, based on the pathohistologic classification developed by Prechtel between 1972 and 1975 (Table 2.6; Prechtel, 1972; Prechtel and Gehm, 1975).

The sonographic features of all grades of fibrocystic disease are extremely varied. If sonographic changes are present, they may take the form of ductal patterns, ductectasia, cysts, ill-defined focal lesions, or architectural distortion (Figs. 2.39–2.41). It is not unusual to find some degree of shadowing behind affected breast tissue. The grade of the disease cannot be established from sonographic criteria. Grade I disease, for example, can mimic a malignant process, while grade III disease may produce no sonographic changes. Recently the claim that the risk of malignant transformation increases with the grade of disease has again been called into question. Indeed, transitions to carcinomatous change may be found in all grades of fibrocystic disease (Fig. 2.42). It can be impossible in some cases to differentiate fibrocystic disease from carcinoma and scar tissue using ultrasound alone (Fig. 2.43). In our own patients (Table 2.7) we find that there is an approximately equal chance of encountering a benign type or a malignant type of sonographic pattern in a fibrocystic breast. These results do not agree with the studies published by Leucht and colleagues (1985): In 131 patients with fibrocystic disease, 96% showed a benign or indifferent pattern and only 4% showed a malignant pattern. This discrepancy may relate to the fact that we examined most of our patients with an automated immersion scanner, whereas Leucht and coworkers used a hand-held real-time scanner exclusively.

Table 2.5. Diffuse benign breast diseases.

Intraductal epithelial proliferations (fibrocystic disease)
Proliferation of myoepithelial cells (sclerosing adenosis)
Proliferation of collagenous connective tissue (fibrosclerosis)

Table 2.6. Classification of fibrocystic breast disease.

Grade	Features
I	Without intraductal epithelial proliferation
II	With intraductal epithelial proliferation but no atypia
III	With intraductal epithelial proliferation and moderate atypia

Developed by Prechtel between 1972 and 1975.

Table 2.7. Ultrasound presentations of fibrocystic disease.

Grade	Unremarkable	Suggestive of benign mass[a]	Suggestive of malignancy	Total
I	2 (8%)	11 (44%)	12 (48%)	25 (100%)
II	8 (19%)	18 (42%)	17 (39%)	43(100%)
III	2 (7%)	9 (31%)	18 (62%)	29 (100%)
Total	12 (12%)	38 (39%)	47 (49%)	97 (100%)

[a] For example, duct ectasia, cysts, etc.

Sclerosing Adenosis and Fibrosclerosis

The lesions of sclerosing adenosis, characterized by a proliferation of myoepithelial cells, are usually diffuse, although tumorlike forms can occur. Like fibrocystic disease, sclerosing adenosis is most commonly seen before the menopause (Figs. 2.44, 2.45). Fibrosclerosis of the breast, marked by a proliferation of collagenous connective tissue, frequently produces a local atrophy of the parenchyma, and its smooth transition with adjacent tissue causes it to be included in the class of diffuse breast diseases (Fig. 2.46).

Although neither sclerosing adenosis or fibrosclerosis has so far demonstrated any link with breast carcinoma (Bässler, 1978), both can simulate malignancy, especially on sonograms.

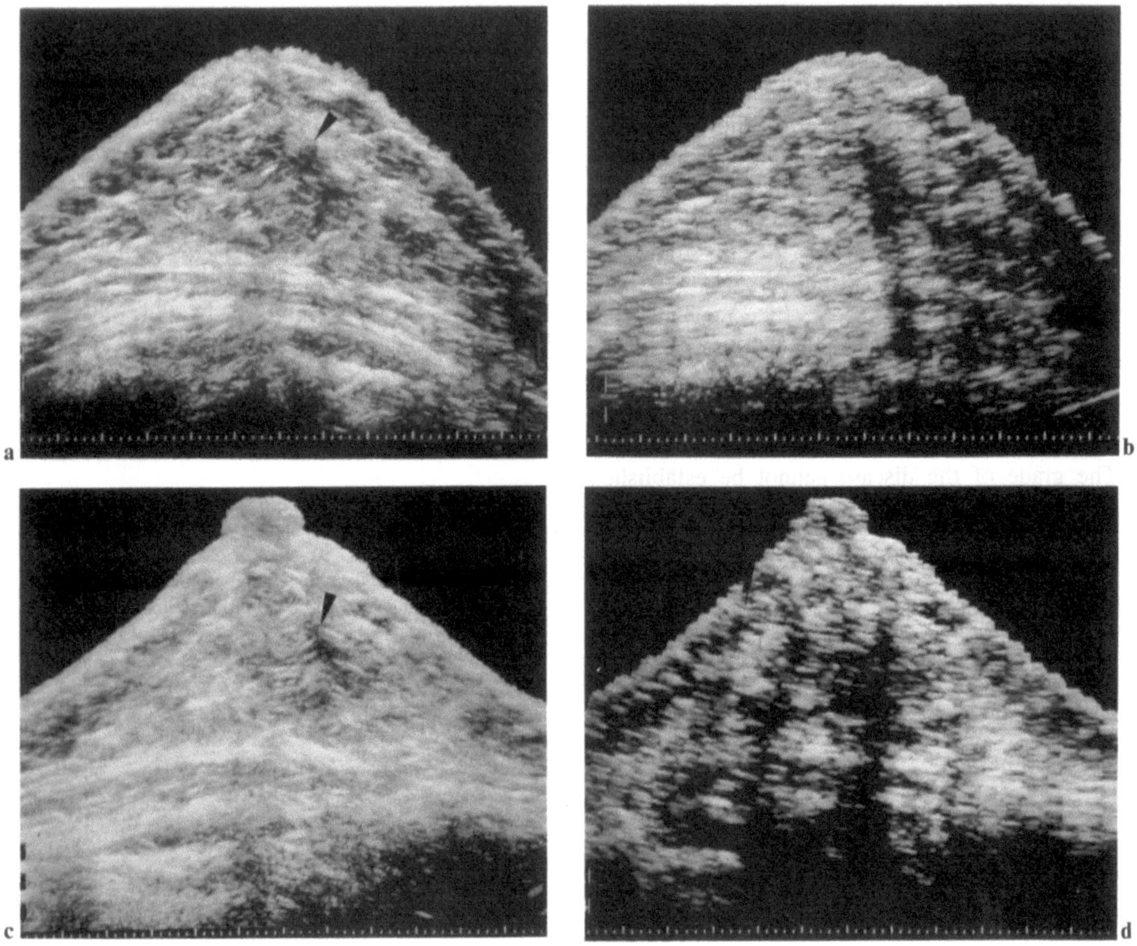

Fig. 2.39a-d. Grade I fibrocystic disease: Architectural distortion with acoustic shadow in a 50-year-old woman with a small nodule in the left lower outer breast quadrant slightly below the nipple

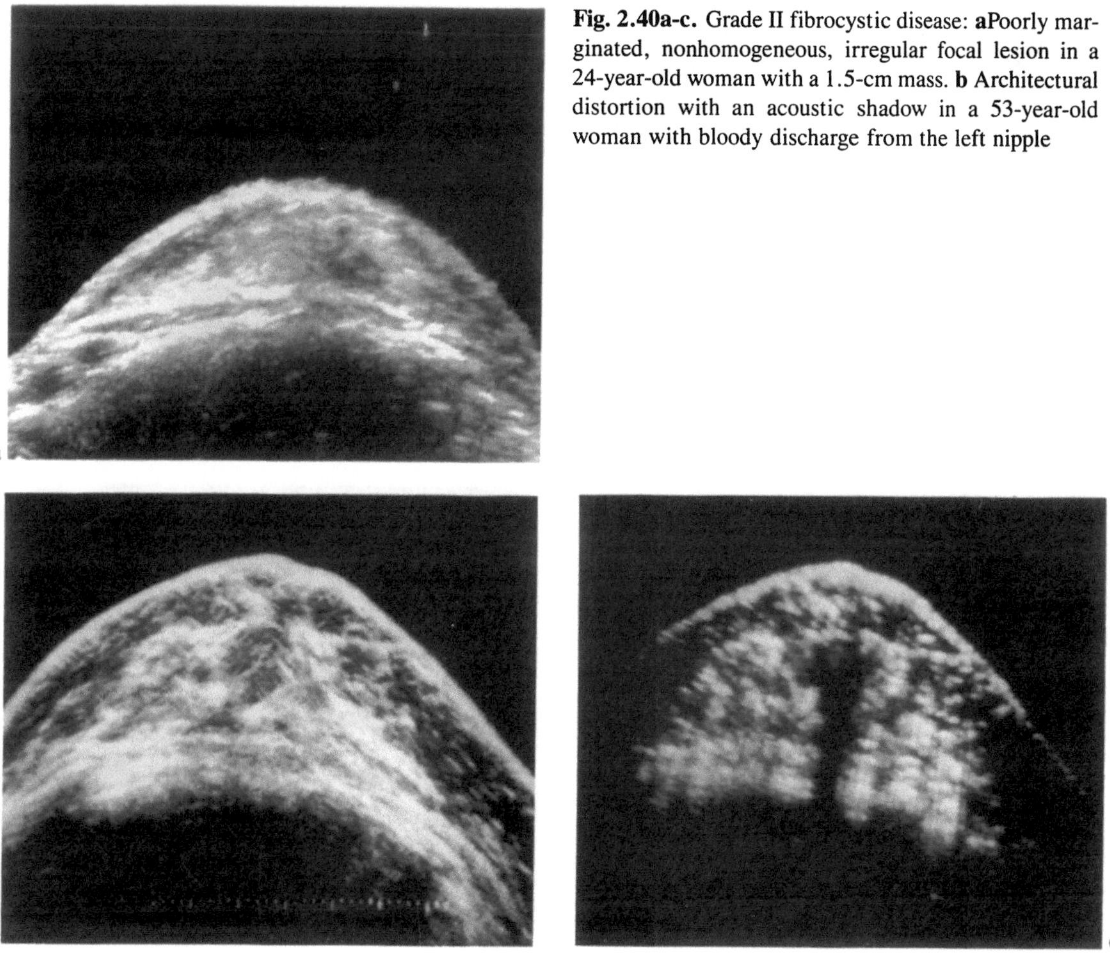

a

b

c

Fig. 2.40a-c. Grade II fibrocystic disease: **a**Poorly marginated, nonhomogeneous, irregular focal lesion in a 24-year-old woman with a 1.5-cm mass. **b** Architectural distortion with an acoustic shadow in a 53-year-old woman with bloody discharge from the left nipple

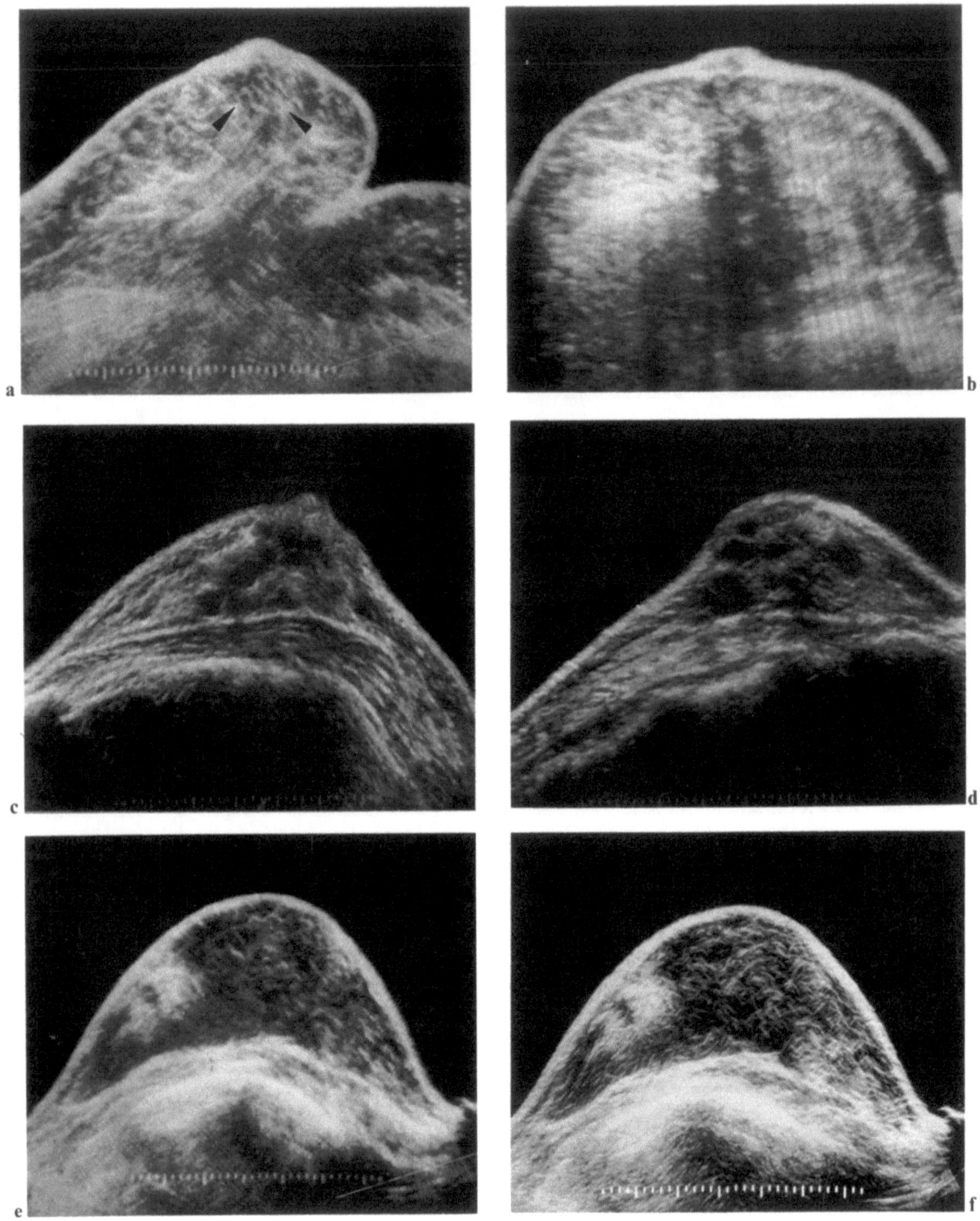

Fig. 2.41a-f. Grade III fibrocystic disease: **a** Area with prominent duct pattern and acoustic shadow in a 63- year-old woman with bloody discharge from the right nipple. **b** Multiple cysts in a 41-year-old woman. **c** Marked hyperechoic structure with a hypoechoic center in a 20-year-old woman with a 1-cm mass in the right breast at 8:30/6 cm (sonograms with soft and hard image display)

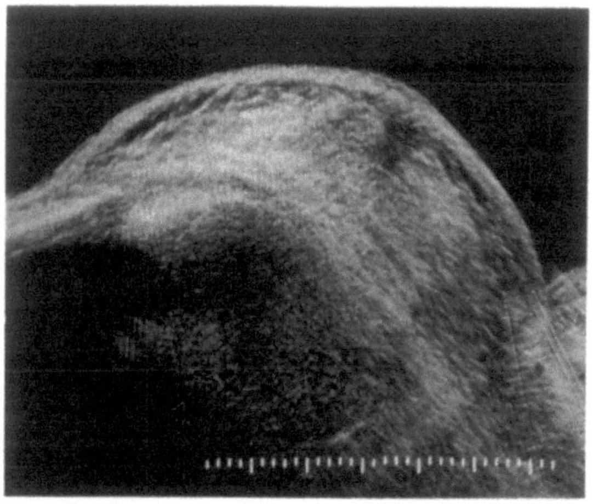
a

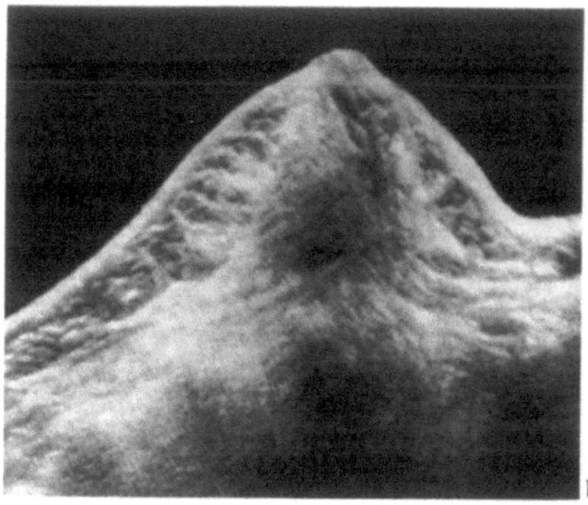
b

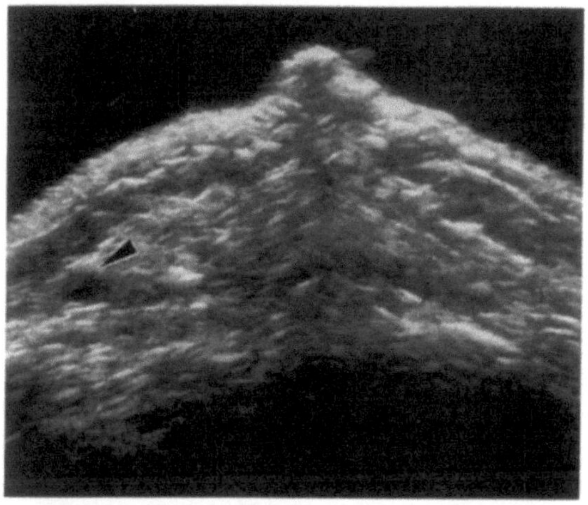
c

Fig. 2.42. a Fibrocystic disease Grade I, and lobular carcinoma in situ (CLIS). **b** Grade II, with CLIS. **c** Grade III, and small invasive carcinoma

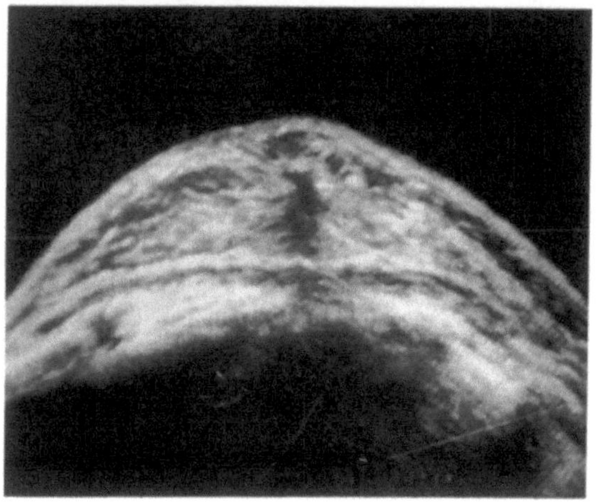

Fig. 2.43. Grade II fibrocystic disease and a scar

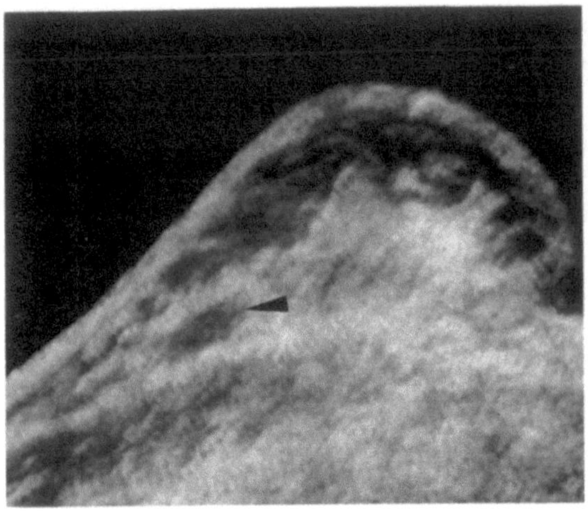

Fig. 2.44. Sclerosing adenosis. **a** Firm bean-size nodule at 1:00 in a 41-year-old woman

a 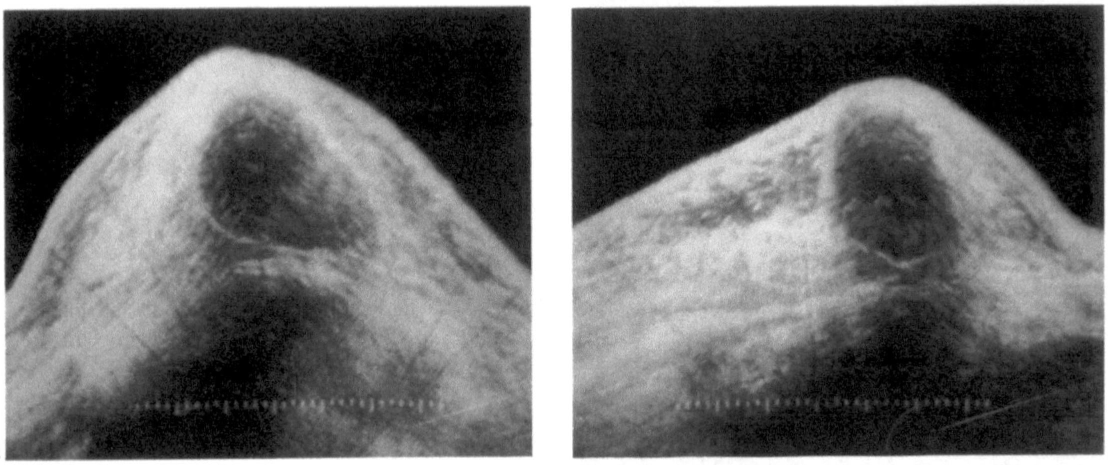 b

Fig. 2.45a,b. Relatively soft 4×4-cm tumorlike mass in the left breast of a 54-year-old woman

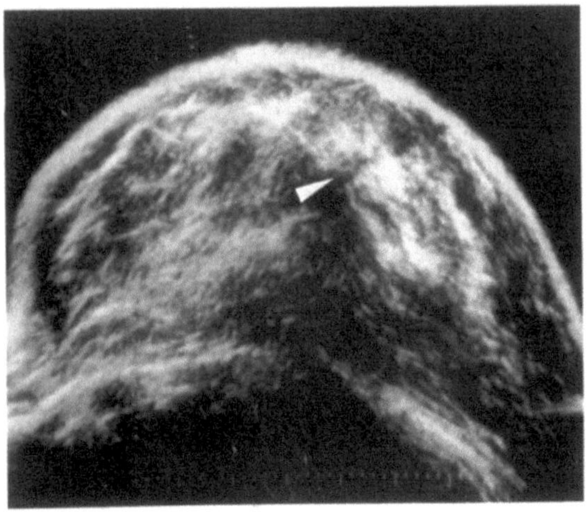

Fig. 2.46. Fibrosclerosis: Firm 2×2-cm mass at 2:00/7 cm in the left breast of a 53-year-old woman

Bibliography

Bässler, R. (1978). Pathologie der Brustdrüse. In Doerr, Seifert, Uehlinger (Eds.), *Spezielle pathologische Anatomie* (Vol. 11). Springer-Verlag, Berlin, Heidelberg, New York.

Callao, J., Hernandez, G., Olloqui, E., Madrid, G., Martinez-Comin, I., Solsona, F. (1977). Ecografia en el diagnóstico del fibroadenoma mamario. *Radiologia 19*, Suppl. 1:71–88.

Cole-Beuglet, C., Soriano, R., Kurtz, A.B., Goldberg, B.B. (1983). Fibroadenoma of the breast: Sonomammography correlated with pathology in 122 patients. *American Journal of Roentgenology 140*:369–375.

Cole-Beuglet, C., Soriano, R., Kurtz, A.B., Meyer, J.E., Kopans, D.B., Goldberg, B.B. (1983). Ultrasound, X-ray mammography, and histopathology of cystosarcoma phylloides. *Radiology 146*:481–486.

Croll, J., Kotevich, J., Tabrett, M. (1982). The diagnosis of benign disease and the exclusion of malignancy in patients with breast symptoms. *Seminars in Ultrasound 3*:38–50.

Cukierfajn, M., Loriaux, Cl., Cattoor, J.P., De Maubeuge, R., Longrée, H., Ardichvili, D. (1980). Granular cell myoblastoma of the breast. *Journal Belge de Radiologie 63*:625–628.

Duda, V. (1982). Ultraschall-Mammographie: Das sonographische Erscheinungsbild anatomischer und pathologischer Strukturen der Mamma unter Anawendung eines Immersionsscanners. Dissertation, University of West Germany, Marburg, pp. 44–71, 86–93.

Eulenburg, R., Hüneke, B., Duda, V., Hackelöer, B.J., Lauth, G., Buchholz, R. (1982). Ultraschallmammographie: Die abszedierende Mastitis und ihre sonographische Differentialdiagnose. *Deutsches Ärzteblatt 79*:31–34/37.

Gairard, B., Dale, G., Gros, Ch. (1976). Echographie et kystes mammaires. *Nucléaire 57*:574–575.

Geißl, G. (1978). Zystenmamma. *Münchner Mediainische Wochenschrift 120*:918.

Heywang, S.H., Lipsit, E.R., Glassman, L.M., Thomas, M.A. (1984). Specificity of ultrasonography in the diagnosis of benign breast masses. *Journal of Ultrasound in Medicine 3*:453–461.

Jaffe, C.C., Rosenfield, A.T., Sommer, G., Taylor, K.J. (1980). Technical factors influencing the imaging of small anechoic cysts by B-scan ultrasound. *Radiology 135*:429–433.

Jellins, J., Hughes, C., Ryan, J., Reeve, T.S., Kossoff, G. (1977). A comparative evaluation of a case of cystosarcoma phylloides: Ultrasound, xeroradiography and thermography. *Radiology 124*:803–804.

Jellins, J., Kossoff, G., Reeve, T.S. (1977). Detection and classification of liquid-filled masses in the breast by grey scale echography. *Radiology 125*: 205–212.

Kalbfleisch, H., Lauth, G., Mühlberger, G., Nitschke, S. (1978). Das Granularzellmyoblastom der weiblichen Brust und seine differentialdiagnostische Abgrenzung gegen das Mammacarcinom. *Radiologe 18*:143–147.

Kleedorfer, D., Pflanzer, D., Pflanzer, K., Kiprov, S., Forchem, K. (1982). Wertigkeit der Ultraschalluntersuchung und sonographische Differentialdiagnose der Mammacyste. *Röntgenblätter 35*:287–294.

Kowand, L.M., Verhulst, L.A., Copeland, C.M., Bose, B. (1984). Epidermal cyst of the breast. *Canadian Medical Association Journal 131*:217–219.

Lang, J., Zana, R., Gairard, B., Dale, G., Gros, Ch. (1978). Ultrasonic absorption in the human breast cyst liquids. *Ultrasound in Medicine and Biology 4*:125–130.

Leucht, W., Rabe, D., Müller, A., von Fournier, D., Humbert, K.D., Schmidt, W. (1985). Verbesserung der präoperativen Abklärung von palpablen, nichtzystischen Prozessen der Mamma durch die Echomammographie. *Ultraschall 6*:19–25.

Prechtel, K. (1972). Beziehungen der Mastopathie zum Mammakarzinom. *Fortschritte der Medicin 90*:43–45.

Prechtel, K., Gehm, O. (1975). Morphologisch faßbare Vorstadien des Mammakarzinoms. *Vehandlung Deutsche Gellschatt Pathologie 59*:498.

Rombaut, M. (1981). Echographie et Kyste Mammaire. *Journale Belge de Radiologie 64*:479–485.

Seymour, E.Q. (1982). Blastomycosis of the breast. *American Journal of Roentgenology 139*:822–823.

Sickles, E.A., Filly, R.A., Callen, P.W. (1984). Benign breast lesions: Ultrasound detection and diagnosis. *Radiology 151*:467–470.

Steinbock, R.T., Stomper, P.C., Meyer, J.E., Kopans, D.B. (1983). The ultrasound appearance of giant fibroadenoma. *Journal of Clinical Ultrasound 11*:451–454.

Volkov, N.A. (1983). Ultrasonographic diagnosis in the treatment of lactation mastitis. *Akush Ginekol 5*:51–53.

3
Malignant Diseases

Breast Carcinoma

In the Federal Republic of Germany, as in the rest of Europe, breast carcinoma is the leading cause of cancer death. In 1981 alone, 12,808 West German women (17.1% of female cancer deaths) died from breast cancer or its sequelae. Approximately 40% of these women died before the age of 65; breast cancer is the leading cause of death in general among women in the 35- to 54-year age group. From 1956 to 1975 the incidence of breast cancer in Central and Western Europe rose at a rate of about 1% annually, resulting in an overall increase of approximately 20% (Becker et al., 1984).

Given these alarming figures, it was natural to place very high expectations on ultrasound as a means for detecting breast carcinoma. But years of experience with breast ultrasound have demonstrated the limitations of the technique and have enabled us to gain a realistic view of its capabilities (Table 3.1).

Of 260 carcinomas studied, ultrasound failed to demonstrate a corresponding focal lesion in 6% of cases (all were T1 cancers). This has been attributed to small tumor size (< 1 cm), masking by adjacent fibrocystic or fibrosclerotic disease, minimal infiltration at the time of the examination, or a multicentric pattern of tumor growth in the form of multiple small nests of tumor cells. Of these undetected carcinomas, 60% occurred in partially involuted breasts, 20% in breasts with high acoustic absorption, and the remaining 20% in homogeneously dense breasts.

The ultrasound features of breast carcinomas are described according to the histopathologic classification of breast carcinomas published by the World Health Organization in 1982 (Table 3.2).

The sonographic features of invasive duct carcinoma are as varied as the distribution of its cellular and connective-tissue elements in histologic sections. The tumor margins can range from smooth to ill defined with "broom-straw" projections and "fir-tree" patterns. Besides being affected by the distribution of cells and connective tissue in the mass, the sonographic pattern can also be affected by the nature of the breast tissue surrounding the lesion. Cellular carcinomas tend to appear as round lesions with relatively ill-defined margins, while stroma-rich carcinomas containing an abundance of connective tissue tend to produce areas of architectural disruption. Fibrocystic or fibrosclerotic changes in proximity to a carcinoma can make the tumor margins appear even less well defined, even in the case of highly cellular cancers. The internal echoes of carcinomas are usually weak, nonhomogeneous, and irregular. Necrotic areas within the tumor can appear anechoic, while calcified areas tend to produce bright echoes.

The most common secondary phenomenon associated with carcinomas is central acoustic shadowing, which may be visible behind the entire mass or portions of it. The shadowing appears to depend on the connective-tissue content of the tumor (Kobayashi, 1979). Shadowing behind the edges of carcinomas apparently results from significant marginal infiltrative growth, and a casual look can create the impression of a benign lesion (Fig. 3.1). Thus, before we take "lateral shadowing" as evidence for a benign mass, we must establish that the entire contour of the tumor is smooth, or that it is surrounded by a "halo" of displaced tissue. Moreover, posterior enhancement may be seen in association with very cellular, slow-growing, or necrotic carcinomas. This occurs

Table 3.1. Efficacy of ultrasound (vs. radiography) in the detection of breast carcinoma.

Smallest carcinoma identified to date as focal lesion	Approx. 5 mm	
Detection of microcalcifications	Apparently detectable with the most modern instruments, but not (yet) identifiable as such in the true sense (see Chap. 5)	
Detection of carcinomas, all stages	Ultrasound:	94%
	X-ray mammography:	95%
Detection of carcinomas ≤1 cm	Ultrasound:	82%
	X-ray mammography:	92%

behind the entire lesion and behind portions of it with approximately equal frequency.

The ultrasound criteria for breast carcinomas may be classified as primary and secondary or as malignancy versus benign mass, as shown in Tables 3.3 and 3.4.

If we compare the sum of the benign mass criteria of a focal lesion (Σ_b) with the sum of its malignancy criteria (Σ_m), we find that 6% of the carcinomas studied have features suggestive of a benign mass ($\Sigma_b > \Sigma_m$), 7% are indifferent ($\Sigma_b = \Sigma_m$), and 87% have features suggestive of malignancy ($\Sigma_b < \Sigma_m$). The advantage of the "'criteria

Table 3.2. Histopathologic classification of breast carcinomas according to the World Health Organization, 1982.

1. Noninvasive carcinomas
   - Intraductal carcinoma
   - Lobular carcinoma in situ (CLIS)
2. Invasive carcinomas
   - Invasive ductal carcinoma (= all carcinomas not otherwise specified, e.g., adenocarcinoma, simple solid carcinoma, scirrhous carcinoma)
   - Invasive ductal carcinoma with a predominant intraductal component
   - Invasive lobular carcinoma
   - Mucinous carcinoma
   - Medullary carcinoma (with little stroma, lymphoid infiltration, and fairly sharp margins)
   - Ductal papillary carcinoma
   - Tubular carcinoma
   - Adenocystic carcinoma
   - Secretory (juvenile) carcinoma
   - Adenocarcinoma with apocrine metaplasia (apocrine carcinoma)
   - Carcinoma with metaplasia:
     - Squamous metaplasia
     - Spindle cell metaplasia
     - Cartilaginous and osseous metaplasia
     - Metaplasia of multiple types
   - Other carcinomas (e.g., lipid-secreting, carcinoidlike, small cell, or signet-ring cell)
3. Paget's carcinoma of the nipple

Adapted from *Histological Typing of Breast Tumors*, 2nd ed., Geneva, World Health Organization 1981 (International Histological Classification of Tumors, No. 2) pp. 15–16.

Table 3.3. Ultrasound criteria for carcinomas, according to frequency.

Criteria	Frequency (%)
Primary	
Margins	
Smooth	1
Halo	0
Ill defined	84
Broom-straw pattern	64
Fir-tree pattern	24
Partially smooth	16
Internal echoes	
Uniform distribution	21
Regular structure	10
Nonuniform distribution	66
Irregular structure	71
Anechoic areas in mass	12
Hyperechoic areas in mass	7
Weak echo pattern	38
Secondary	
Posterior acoustic enhancement	
Behind portions of mass	10
Behind entire mass	11
Behind entire mass on both planes	7
Acoustic shadowing	
Lateral	0
Central	74
Central on both planes	56

Table 3.4. Ultrasound criteria for carcinomas grouped according to benign mass and malignancy criteria.

Benign mass	
Smooth margins	1
Halo	0
Lateral shadowing	0
Uniform distribution of internal echoes	21
Regular structure of internal echoes	10
Enhancement behind entire mass	11
Enhancement on both planes	7
Malignant	
Ill-defined margins	84
Broom-straw pattern	64
Fir-tree pattern	24
Nonuniform distribution of internal echoes	66
Irregular structure of internal echoes	71
Central acoustic shadow	74
Central acoustic shadow on both planes	56

addition" method is that it does not place undue emphasis on individual interpretive criteria, and it yields very good results in comparison with both other authors' results and other methods of examination such as palpation and radiography. A detailed evaluation of this method is presented in Chapter 5.

If we disregard the evaluation of individual criteria or their addition by category and instead look at the combinations of criteria that are seen, we find that recurring patterns emerge. The smaller carcinomas with partially smooth margins, weak internal echoes, and an absence of secondary phenomena present the least characteristic picture in this regard (Figs. 3.2–3.4). There are any number of gradations from this type to the poorly marginated round lesion with nonhomogeneous, irregular internal echoes and absent or subtle secondary phenomena (Figs. 3.5–3.8). As the tumor margins become less well defined, the echoes from the focal lesion tend to become weaker, especially in smaller carcinomas. Posterior attenuation and central shadowing may be seen in association with ill-defined lesions also (Fig. 3.9). Experience has shown that acoustic shadowing is seen more frequently on immersion scans of the freely suspended breast than on hand-held real-time scans taken with compression (Figs. 3.10–3.13). This does not mean, however, that manual scans are incapable of demonstrating acoustic shadowing (Fig. 3.14). The ability to elicit this secondary phenomenon, as well as acoustic enhancement, depends not just on the sonographic technique (examination method and transducer frequency) and the tumor itself, but also on the location of the tumor in the breast (superficial or deep, central or peripheral) and on the general structure of the glandular tissue.

The larger image field and lack of compression with the immersion method make it easier in many cases to assess the behavior of tumor in relation to its environment, that is, to distinguish between a "pushing" and an "infiltrating" type of growth.

Water-path coupling of the transducer is necessary for the visualization of skin changes, and the free immersion technique is optimum. Tumor-related bulging, flattening, or retraction of the skin is readily demonstrated (Fig. 3.16a,b). Carcinomatous lymphangiosis or ulceration of the skin will loosen or disrupt the normally uniformly hyperechoic cutaneous layer (Fig. 3.16c,d).

Pectoralis infiltration is demonstrated most clearly with a manual real-time scanner. The accompanying compression shortens the path of the beam to the pectoral fascia, and there is no sector overlap, as in a compound immersion scan, that might obscure the details of deeper structures. Pectorialis infiltration appears sonographically as an area of fascial disruption that is continuous with the primary tumor (Fig. 3.17).

Multiple focal lesions associated with multicentric tumor growth can be resolved equally well by the immersion and manual real-time techniques (Fig. 3.18a-f). Compared with radiographs and other summation images, the cross-sectional image produced by ultrasound can even be advantageous in identifying lesions that are separate from one another (Fig. 3.18g).

Anechoic areas that are noted in association with breast carcinomas may represent areas of tumor necrosis, hemorrhage, or even intracystic carcinoma (Figs. 3.19–3.21).

Breast carcinomas that show a specific type of tissue differentiation (mucinous, medullary, papillary, tubular, or adenocystic growth, or carcinomas with metaplasia) are uncommon. Evidence to date indicates that these tumors tend to exhibit benign or indifferent sonographic features (Figs. 3.22–3.32).

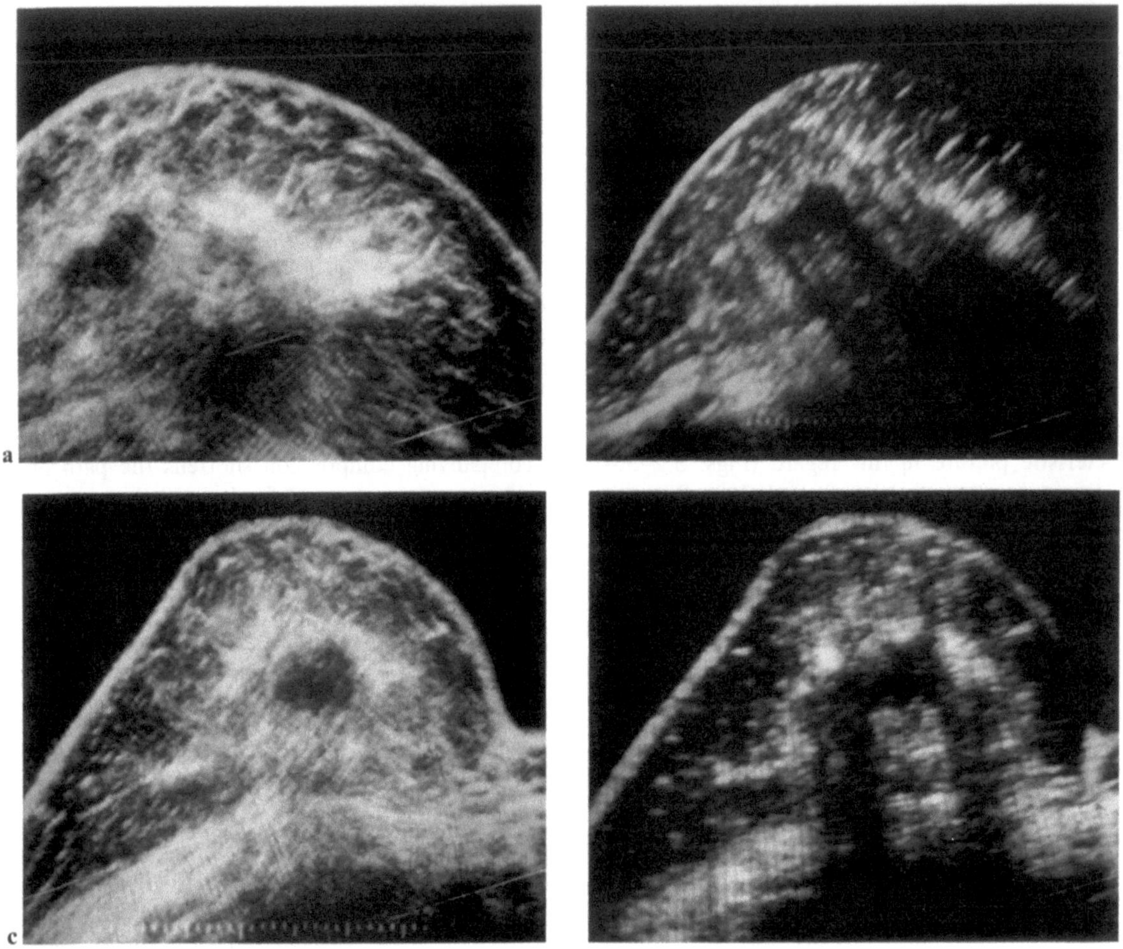

a b c d

Fig. 3.1a-d. 2.5-cm simple solid carcinoma in a 55-year-old woman. The rounded shape of the mass and the shadowing at its edges can easily create the impression a benign mass.

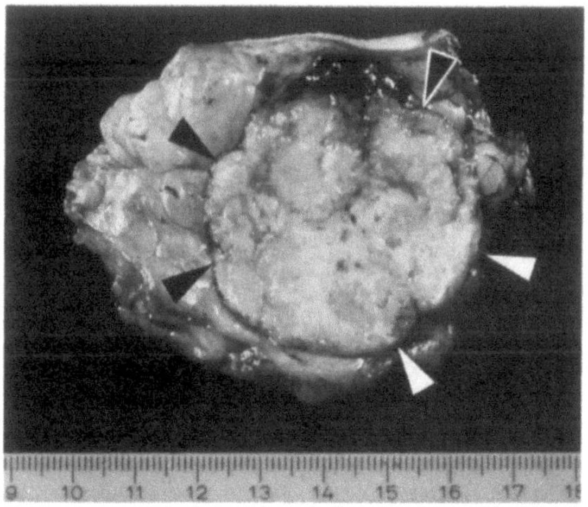

Fig. 3.2. Gross appearance of a cellular carcinoma

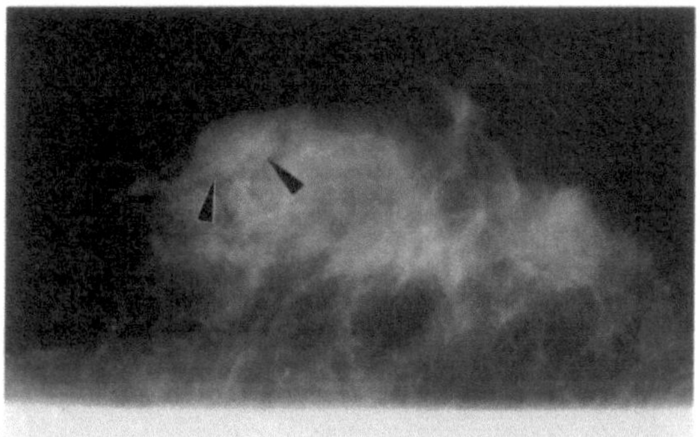

a

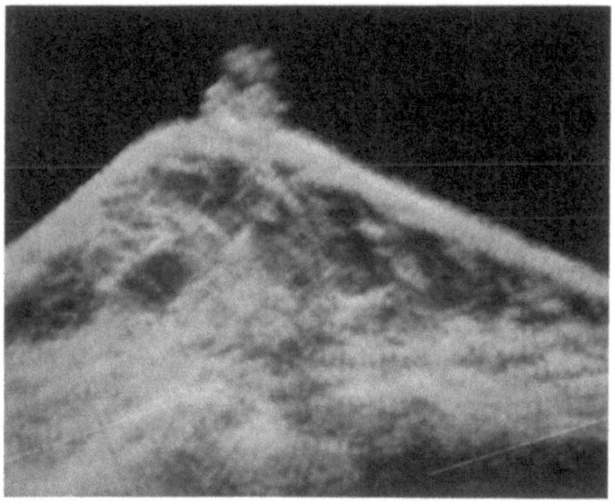

b

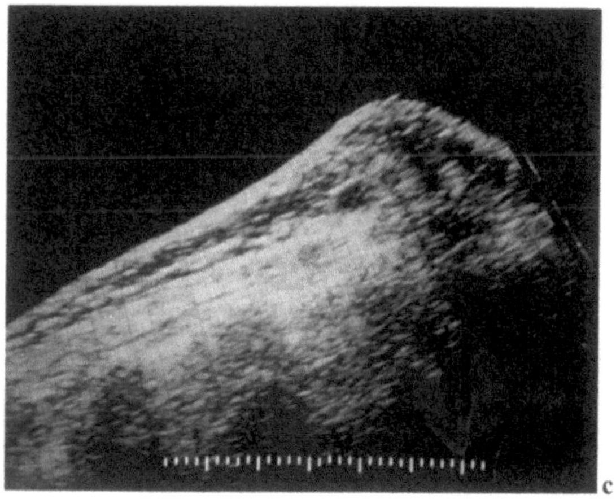

c

Fig. 3.3a-c. Radiograph (**a**) and sonograms (**b,c**) of a cellular (solid) carcinoma in a 57-year-old woman

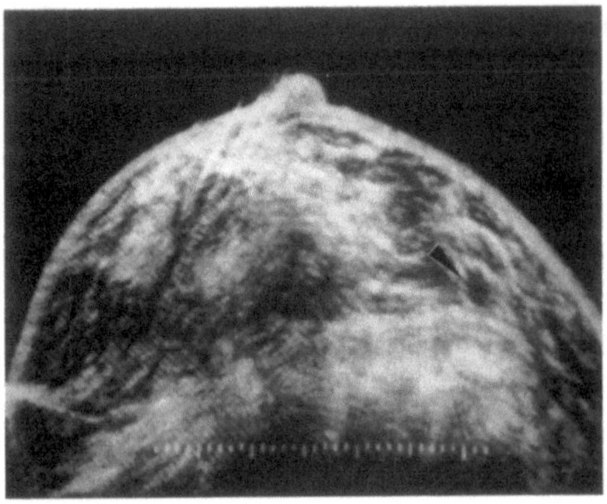

Fig. 3.4. 1.4-cm glandular-cribriform carcinoma in a 39-year-old woman with a 2.5-cm mass in the left upper outer breast quadrant

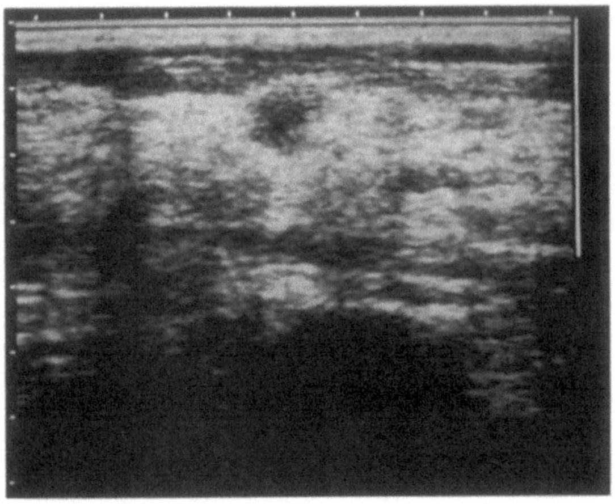

Fig. 3.5. 1.6-cm cribriform-papillary carcinoma in a 47-year-old woman with a 1.5-cm mass in the right breast at 8:30/4.5 cm

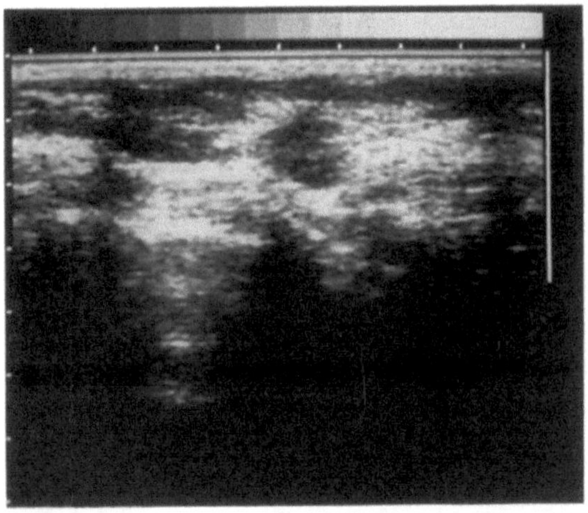

Fig. 3.6. 2.2-cm cribriform carcinoma in a 75-year-old woman with a 2-cm mass in the left breast at 11:00/3 cm

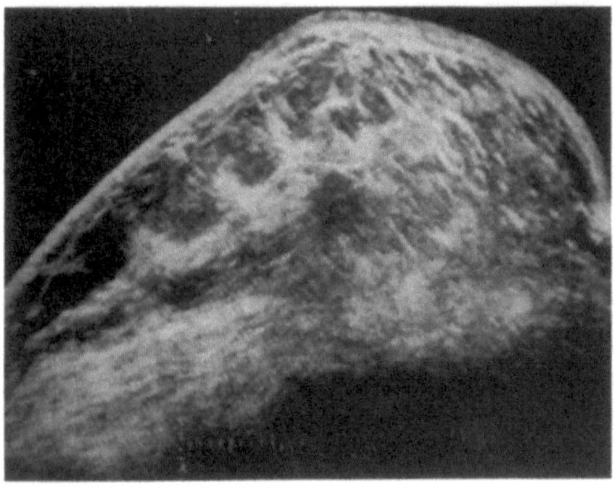

Fig. 3.7. 4-cm solid carcinoma in a 65-year-old woman with a 5-cm mass in the right breast at 8:00

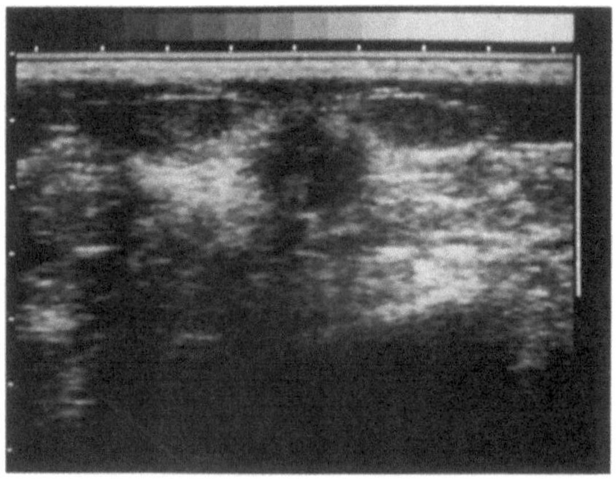

Fig. 3.8. 2.5-cm scirrhous carcinoma in a 46-year-old woman with a 2-cm mass in the right breast at 1:30/2 cm

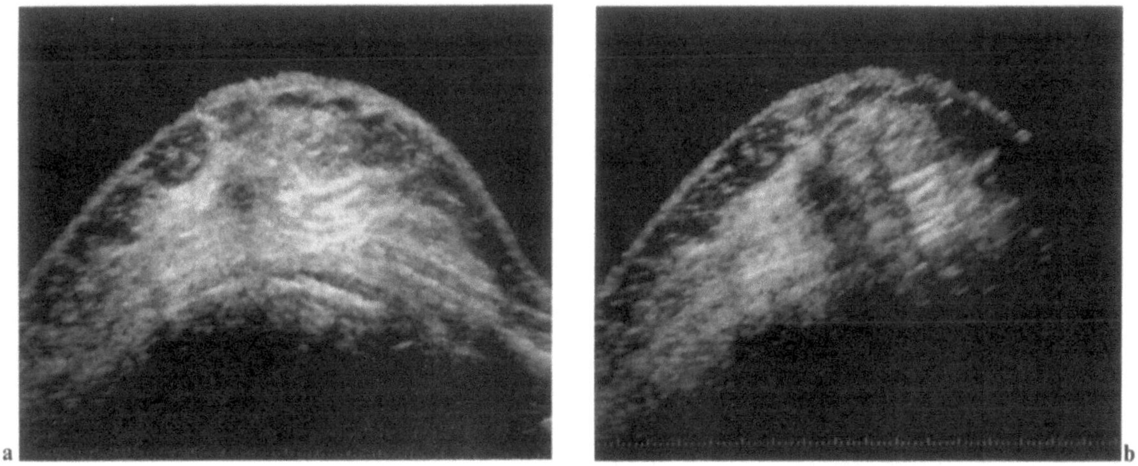

Fig. 3.9a,b. 1.5-cm solid carcinoma in a 53-year-old woman with a 2-cm mass in the right breast at 7:30/3 cm

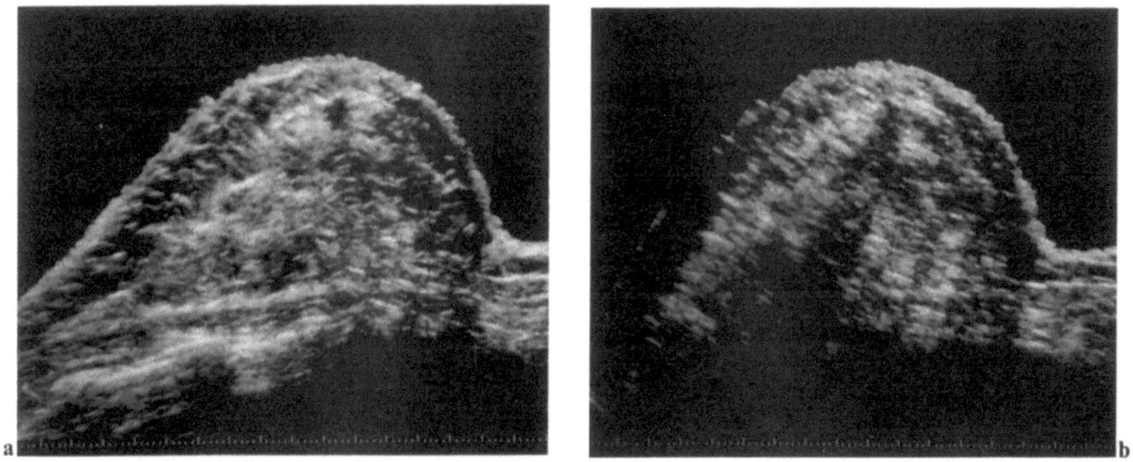

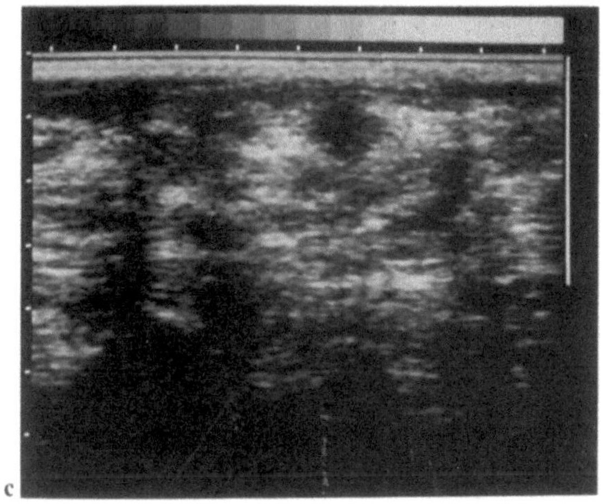

Fig. 3.10a-c. 1.3-cm solid carcinoma with central hyalinosis and marked fibrosclerosis in a 37-year-old woman with a firm 2-cm mass in the left breast at 9:00/2 cm

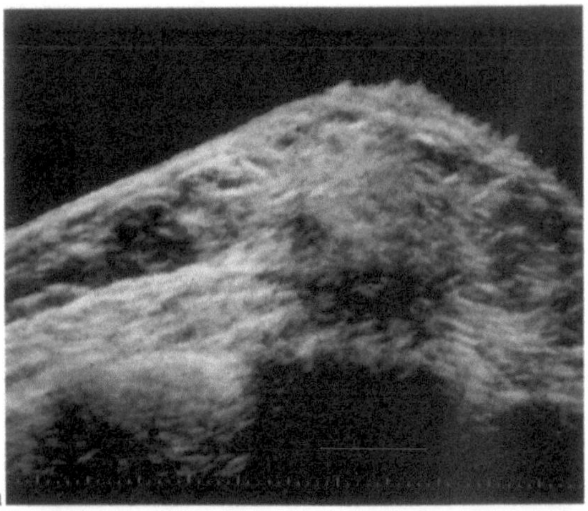

a

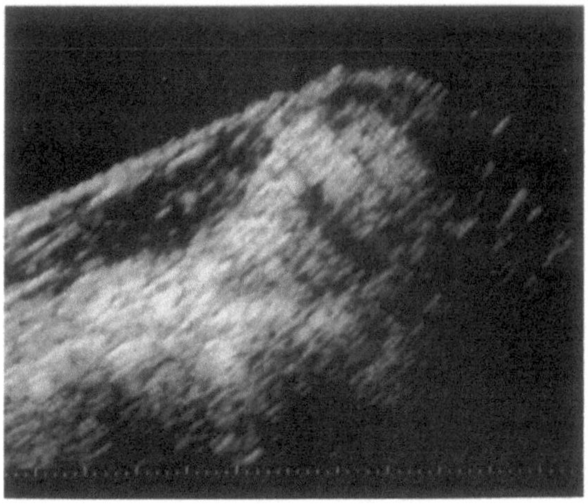

b

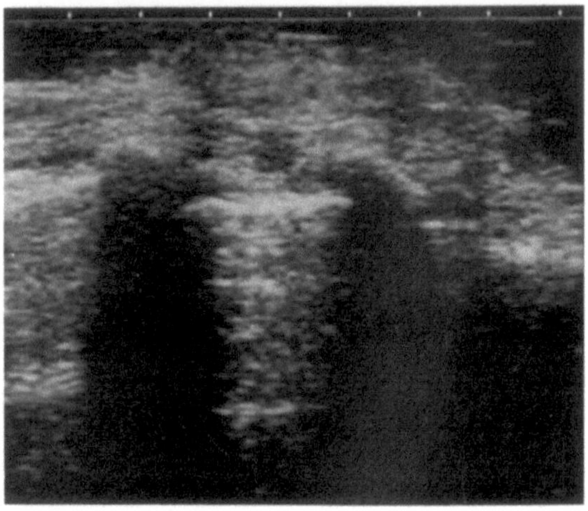

c

Fig. 3.11a-c. Small scirrhous carcinoma in a 45-year-old woman with a pea-size nodule in the right breast at 11:30/2.5 cm

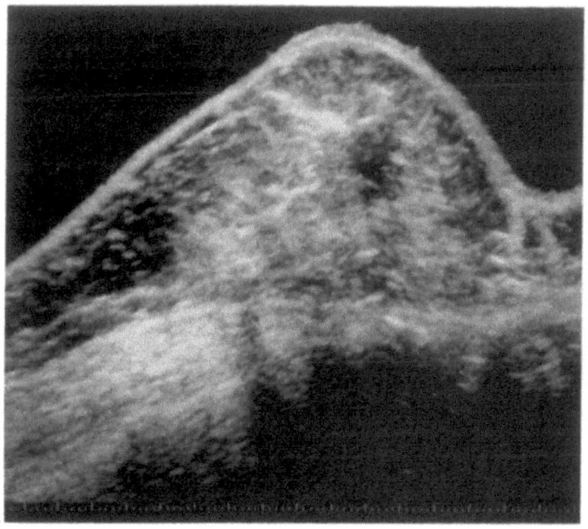

a

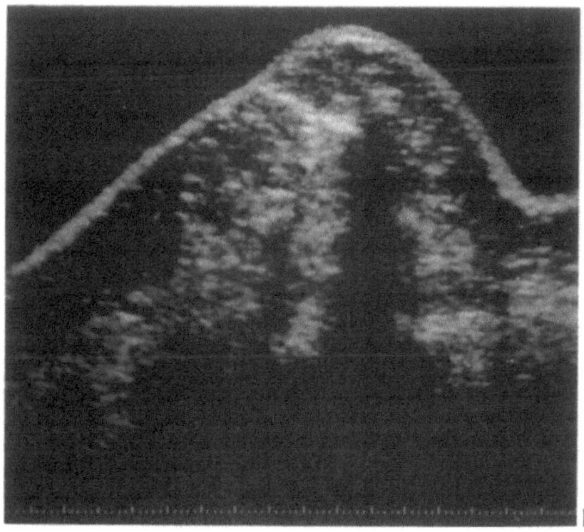

b

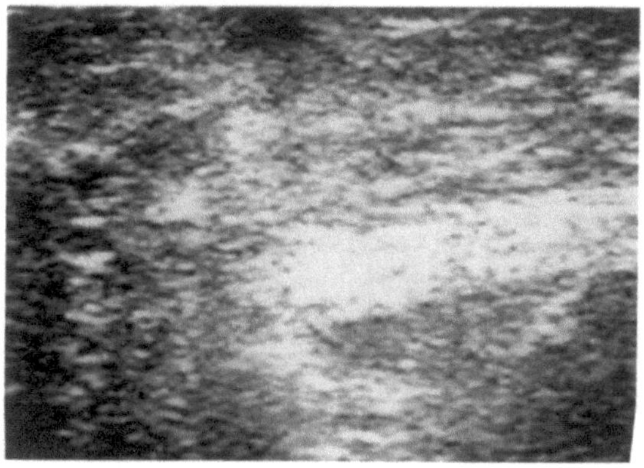

c

Fig. 3.12a-c. 2.9-cm solid-scirrhous carcinoma in a 47-year-old woman with a 3.5-cm mass in the left breast at 11:00/4 cm

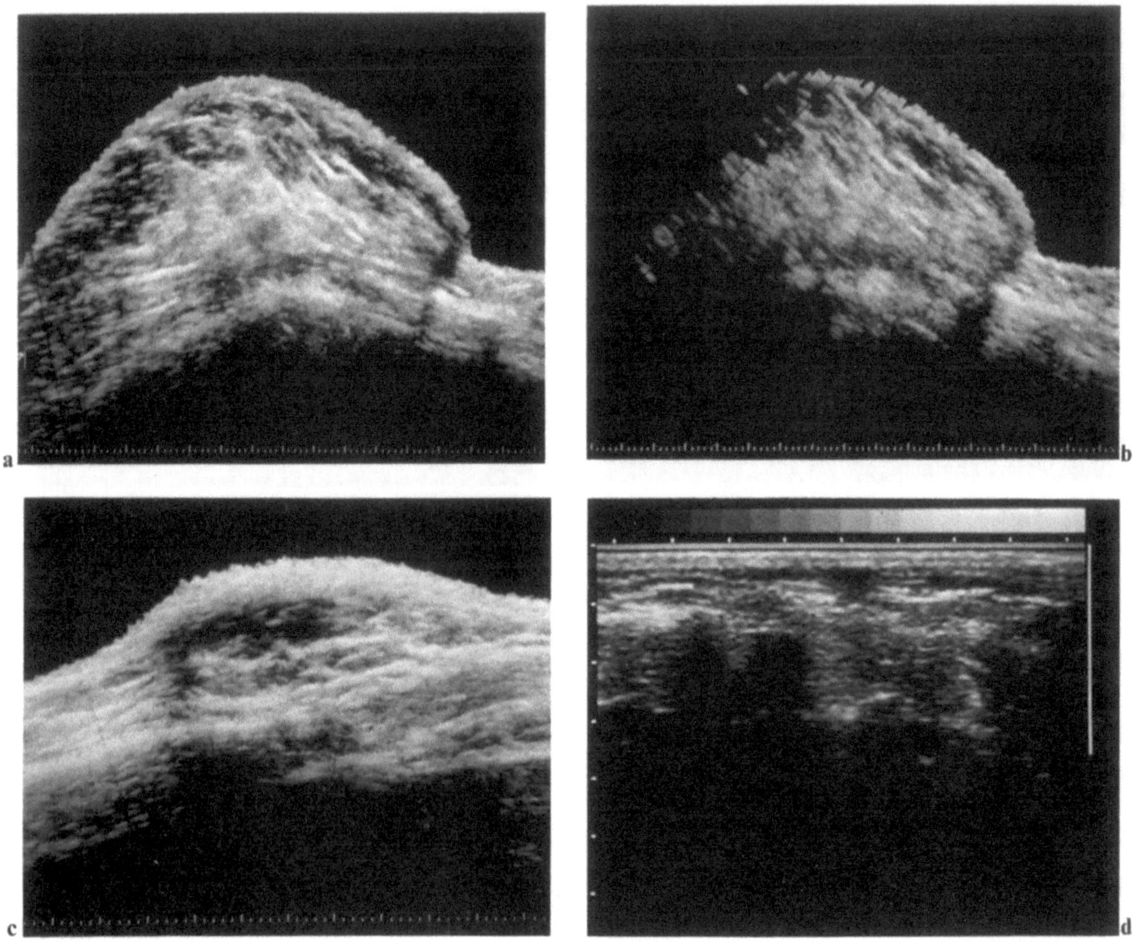

Fig. 3.13a-d. 1-cm scirrhous carcinoma in a 48-year-old woman with a firm 3-cm mass in the right breast at 2:30/11 cm

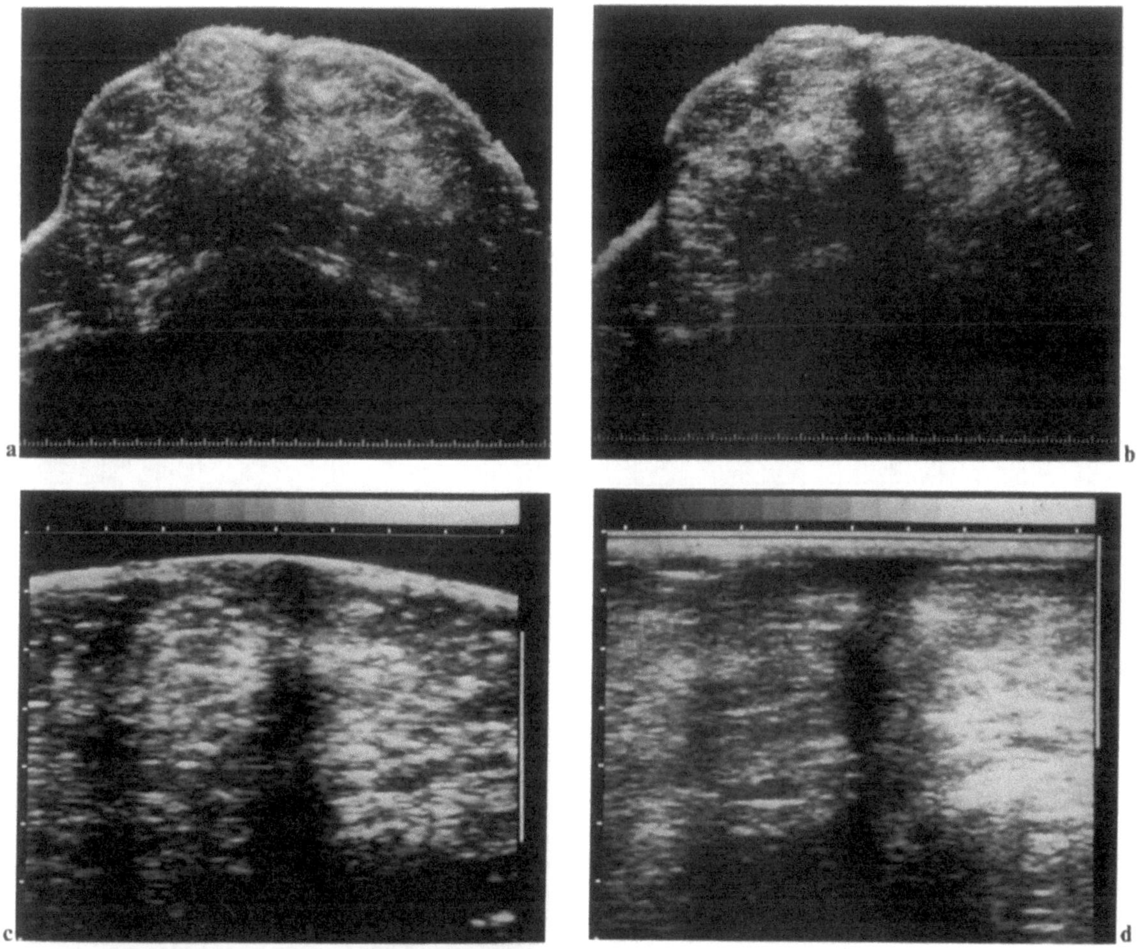

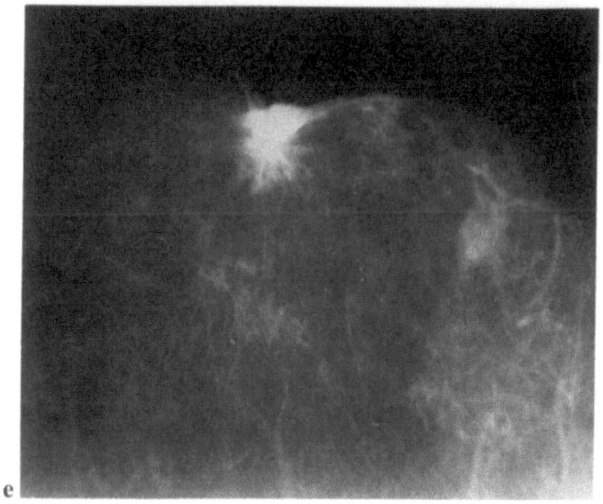

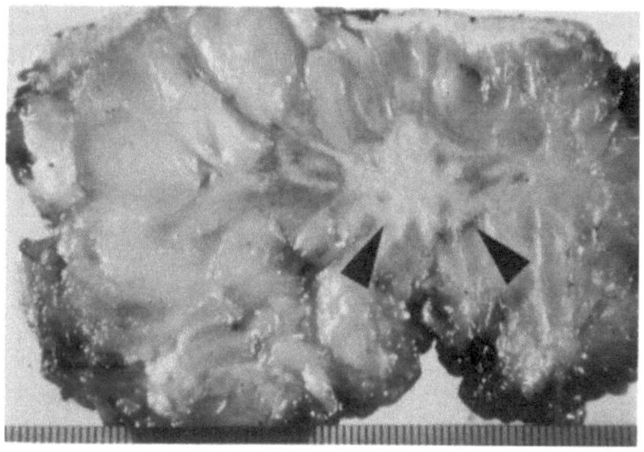

Fig. 3.14a-e. Sonograms and radiograph of a stroma-rich (scirrhous) carcinoma in a 64-year-old woman

Fig. 3.15. Gross appearance of a stroma-rich carcinoma

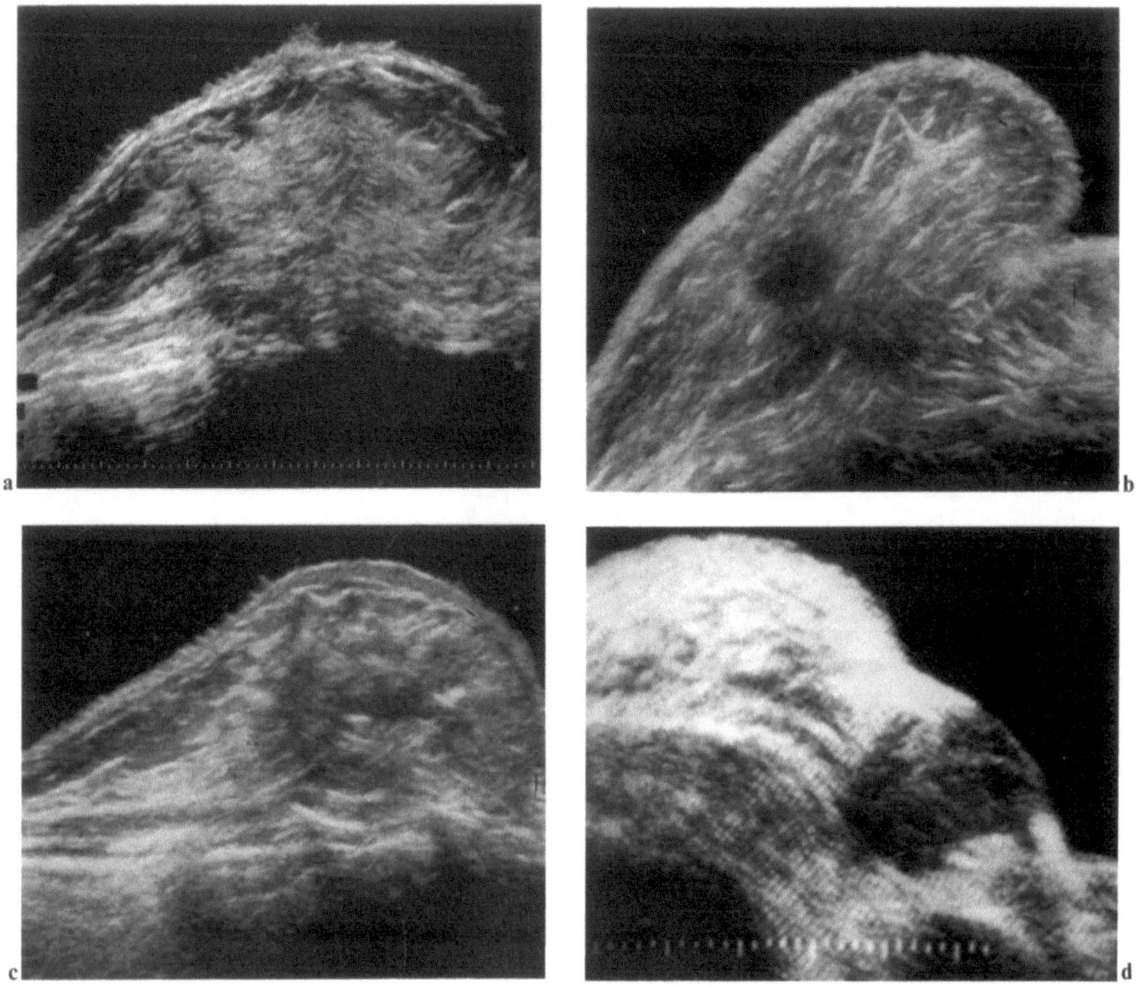

Fig. 3.16a-d. Skin changes associated with breast carcinoma. **a** Bulging. **b** Retraction. **c** Carcinomatous lymphagiosis. **d** Ulceration

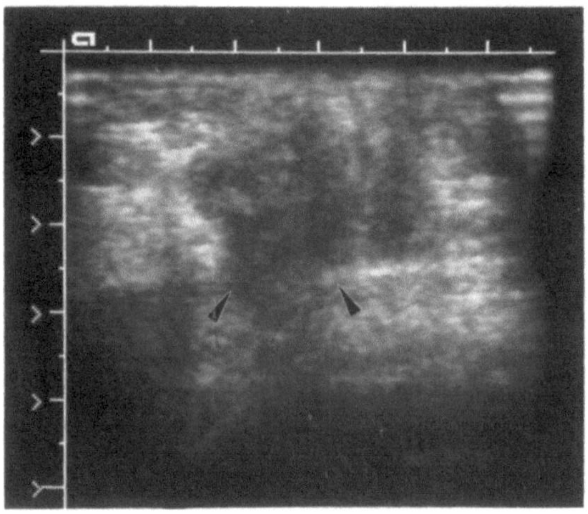

Fig. 3.17. Pectoralis infiltration

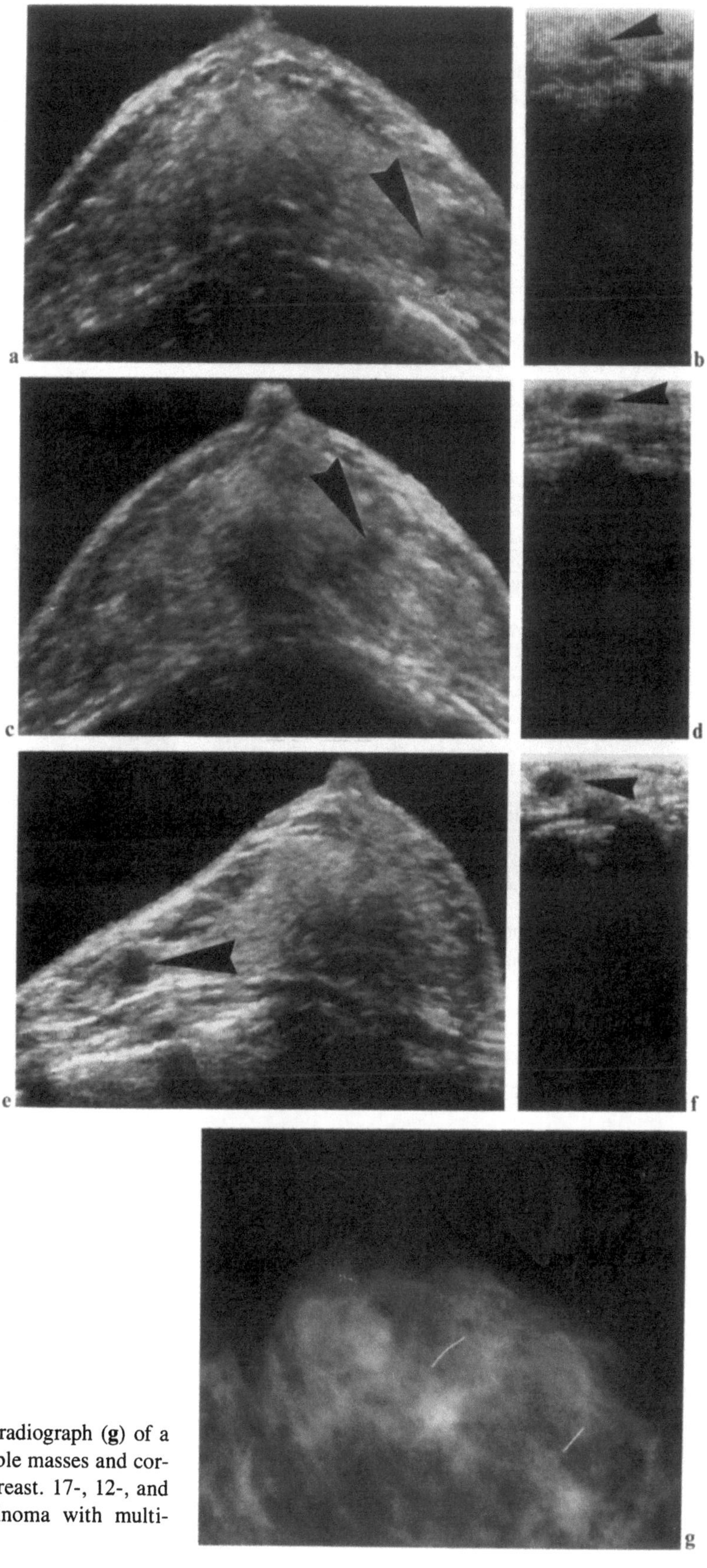

Fig. 3.18a-g. Sonograms (**a**–**f**) and radiograph (**g**) of a 32-year-old woman with three palpable masses and corresponding focal lesions in the left breast. 17-, 12-, and 9-mm foci of solid-scirrhous carcinoma with multicentric growth

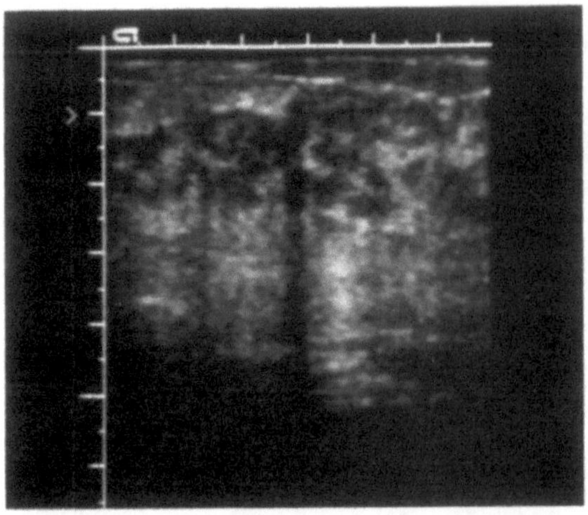

Fig. 3.19. Extensive partly fibrotic, partly necrotic carcinoma in a 59-year-old woman. Note the adjacent zones of acoustic shadowing and posterior acoustic enhancement

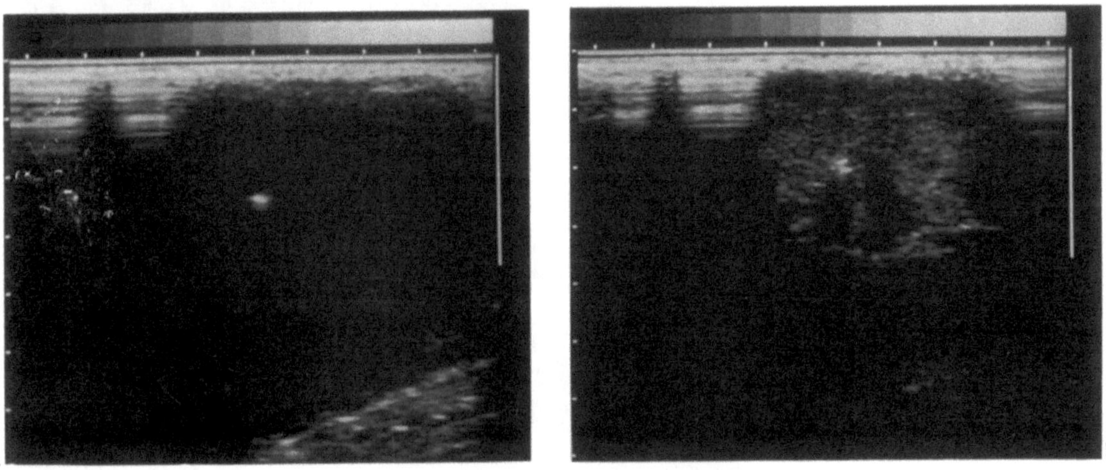

a b

Fig. 3.20a,b. Carcinoma with internal bleeding in a 76-year-old woman before (**a**) and after (**b**) needle aspiration of 60 ml of blood-tinged fluid. The tip of the aspirating needle appears as a bright echo

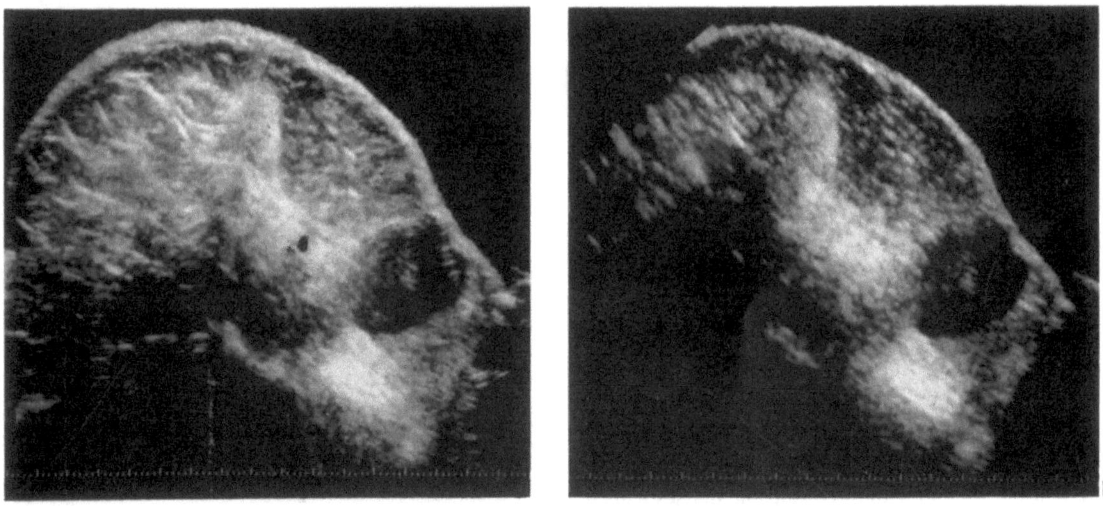

a b

Fig. 3.21a,b. Infiltrating intracystic carcinoma in a 78-year-old woman with a large mass in the left breast. There is obvious skin fixation by the underlying tumor

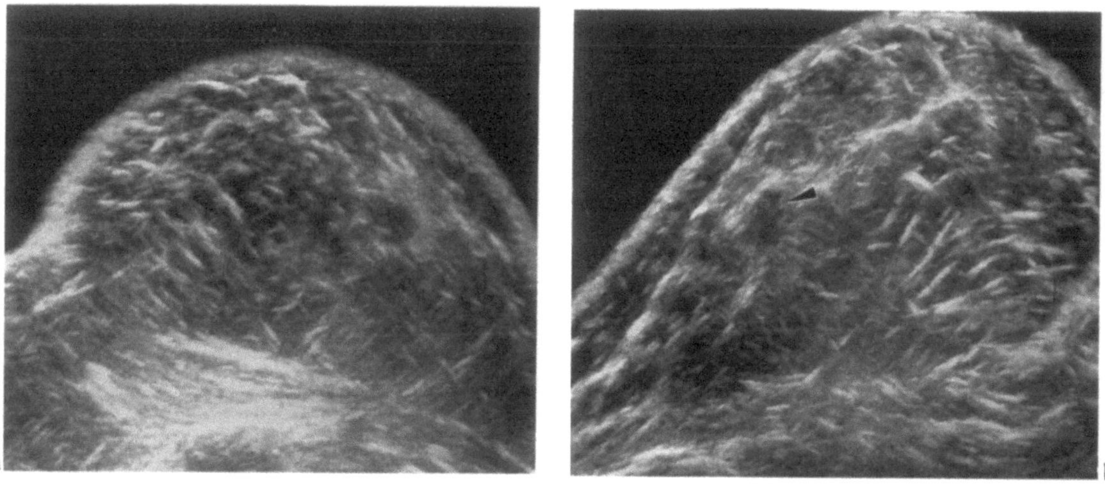

Fig. 3.22a,b. 1.5-cm mucinous carcinoma in a 60-year-old woman with a firm 2-cm mass at 1:30/7 cm in the left breast

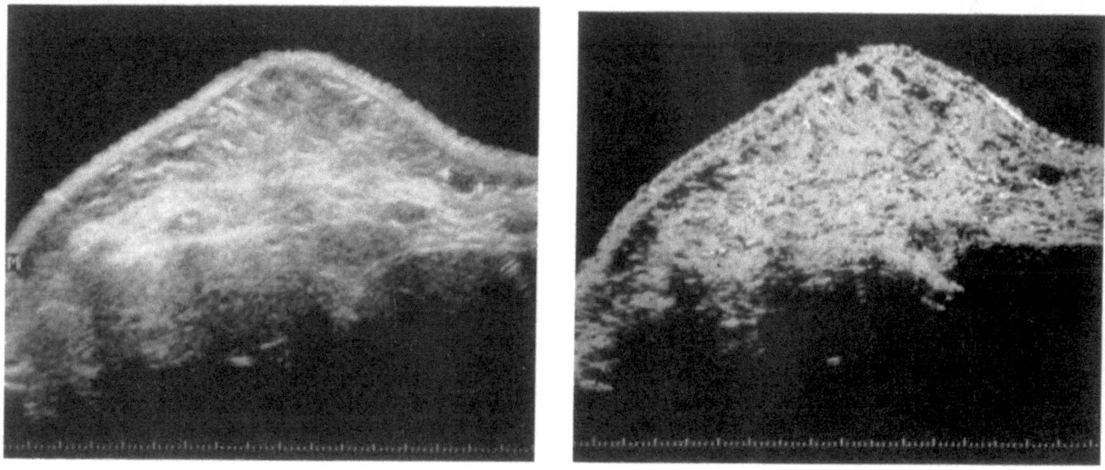

Fig. 3.23a,b. 1-cm mucinous carcinoma in a 64-year-old woman with a firm 1.5-cm mass at 5:00/6 cm in the right breast; normal and postprocessed images

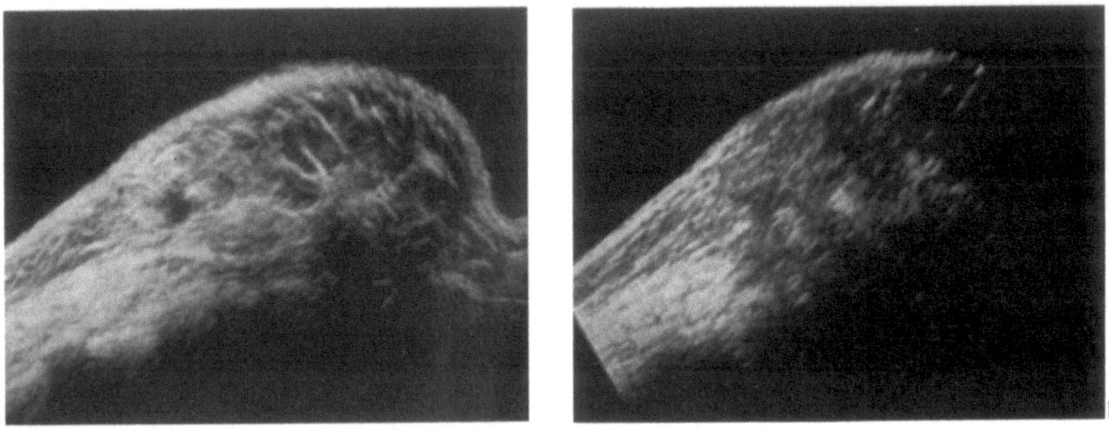

a b

Fig. 3.24a,b. 1.6-cm medullary carcinoma in a 71-year-old woman with a firm 2-cm mass at 12:00/6 cm in the left breast

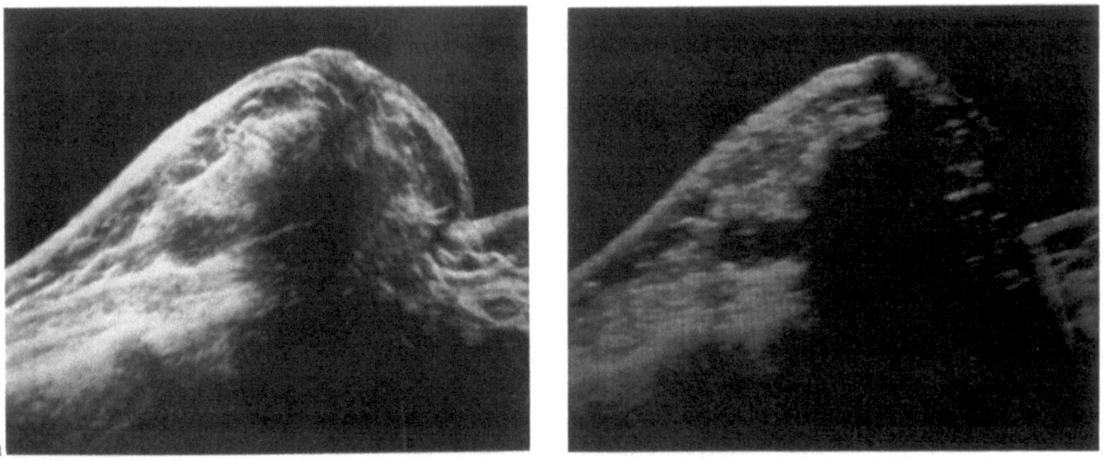

a b

Fig. 3.25a,b. 2.6-cm medullary carcinoma in a 44-year-old woman with a 3-cm mass at 11:30/6 in the left breast

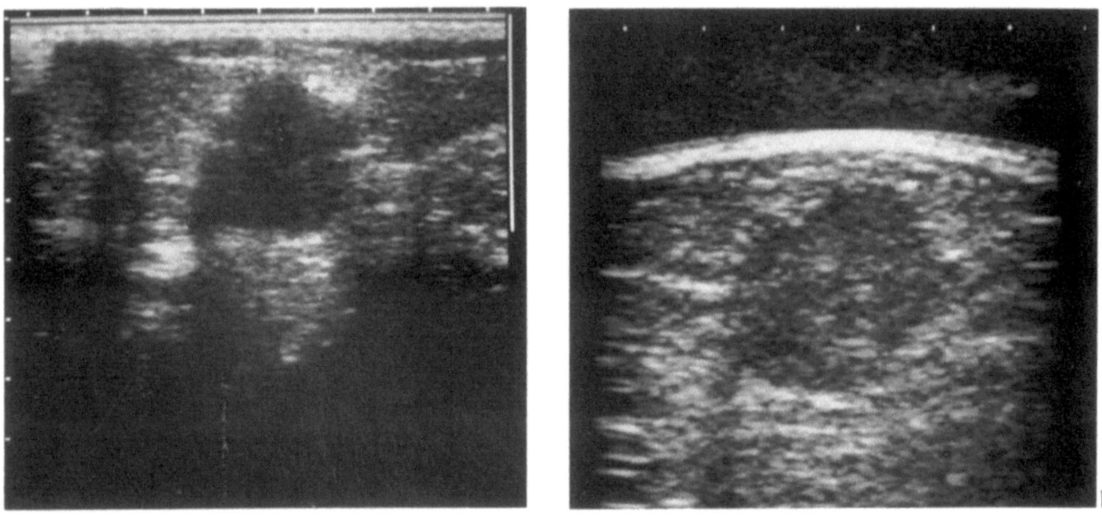

a b

Fig. 3.26a,b. 3-cm medullary carcinoma in a 60-year-old woman with a firm 4-cm mass in the right upper outer breast quadrant

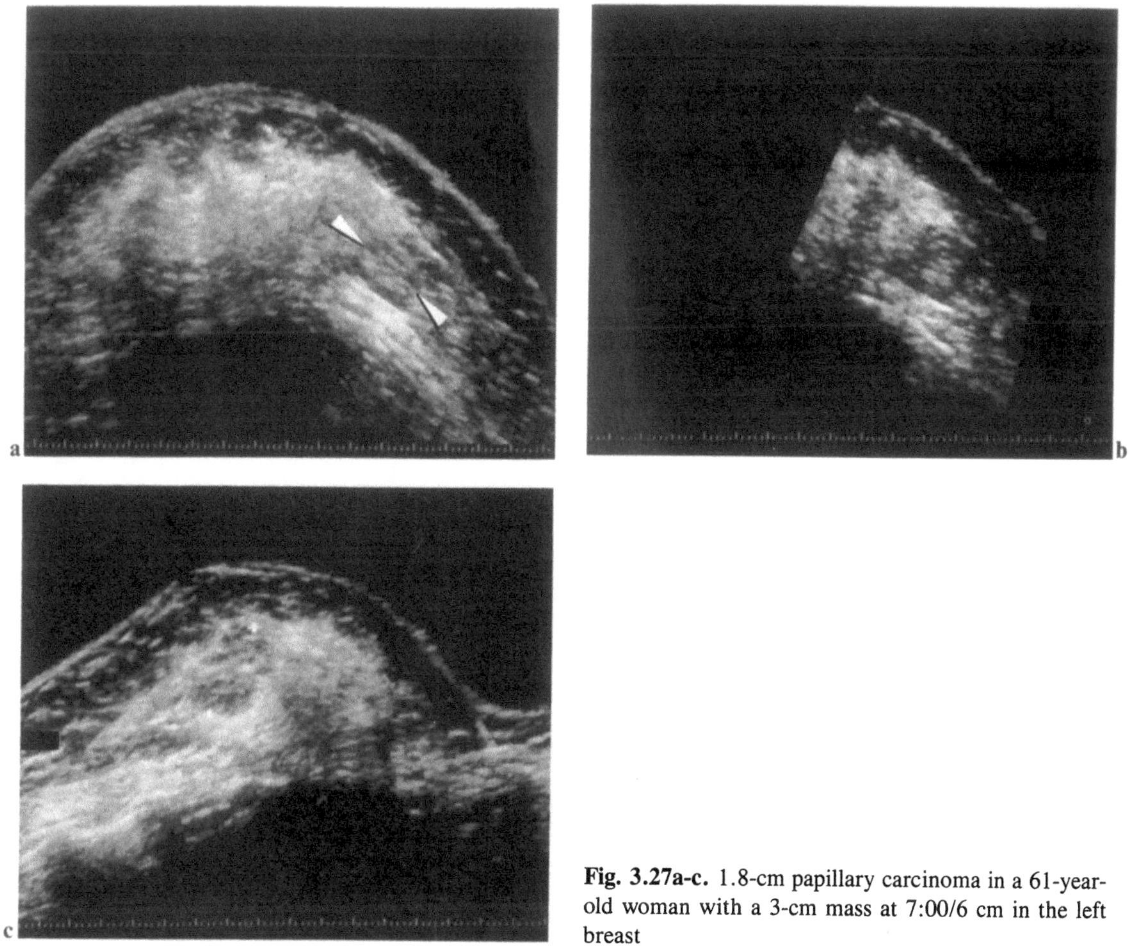

Fig. 3.27a-c. 1.8-cm papillary carcinoma in a 61-year-old woman with a 3-cm mass at 7:00/6 cm in the left breast

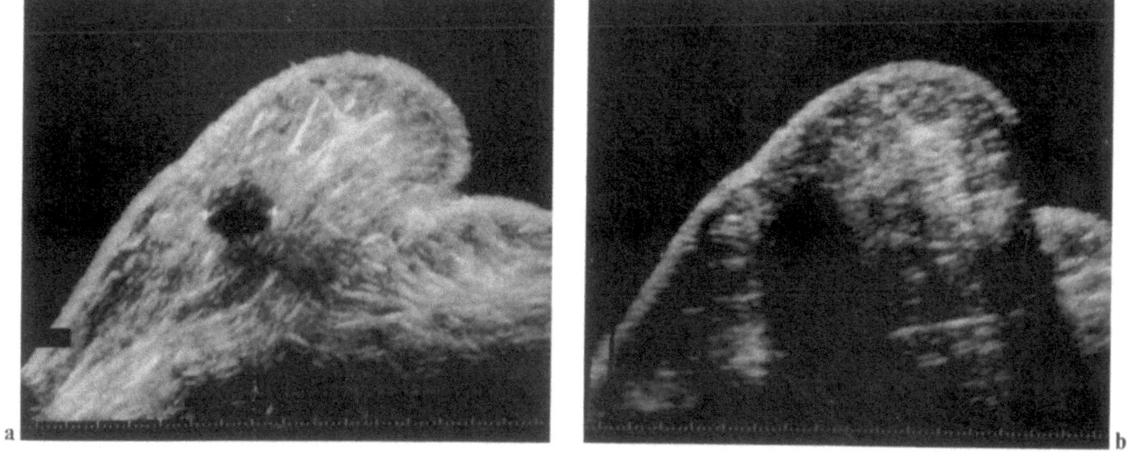

Fig. 3.28a,b. 3-cm papillary carcinoma in a 74-year-old woman with a firm 3.5-cm at 2:30/7 cm in the right breast

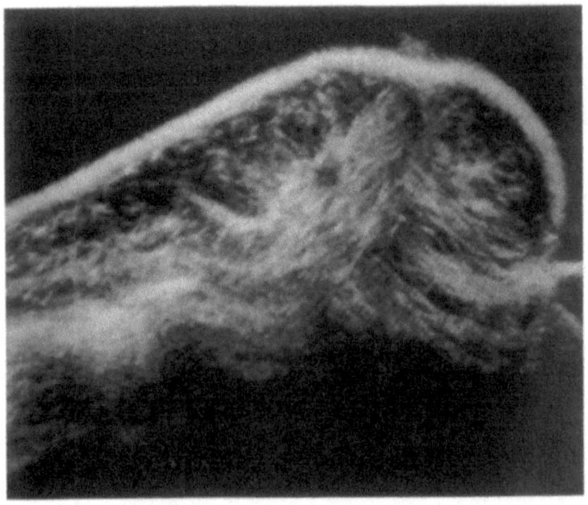

Fig. 3.29. 1.2-cm tubular carcinoma in a 57-year-old woman with a 1.5-cm mass at 11:30/4.5 cm in the left breast

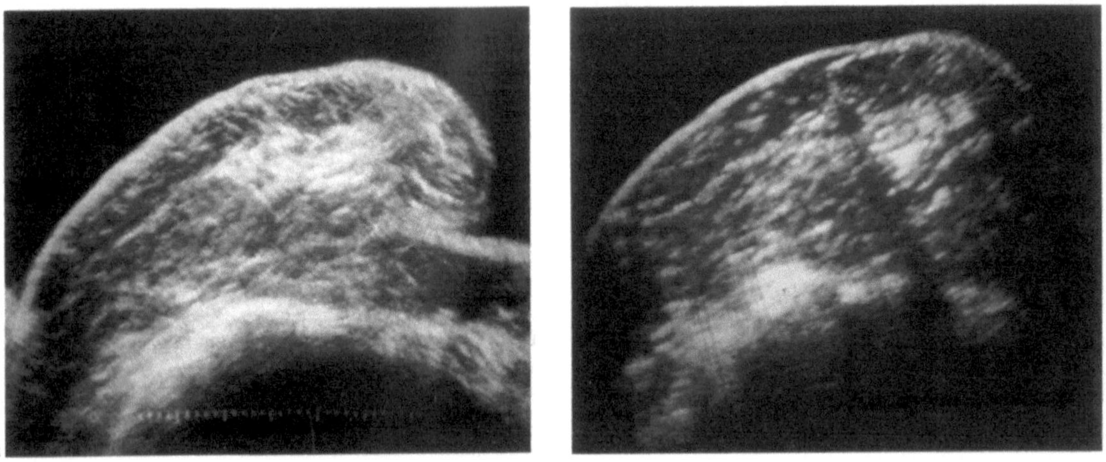

Fig. 3.30a,b. 1-cm tubular carcinoma in a 72-year-old woman with a density at 11:00/1.5 cm in the right breast

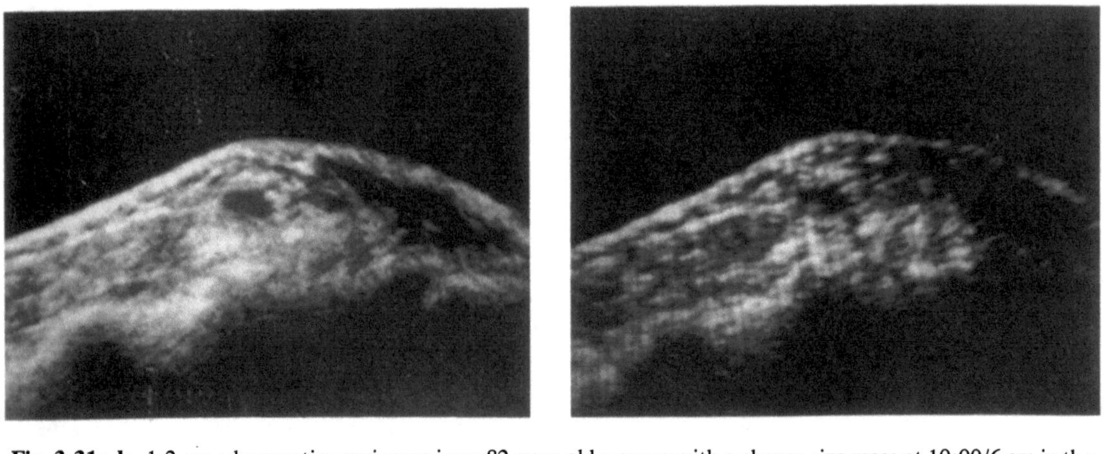

Fig. 3.31a,b. 1.2-cm adenocystic carcinoma in an 82-year-old woman with a cherry-size mass at 10:00/6 cm in the right breast

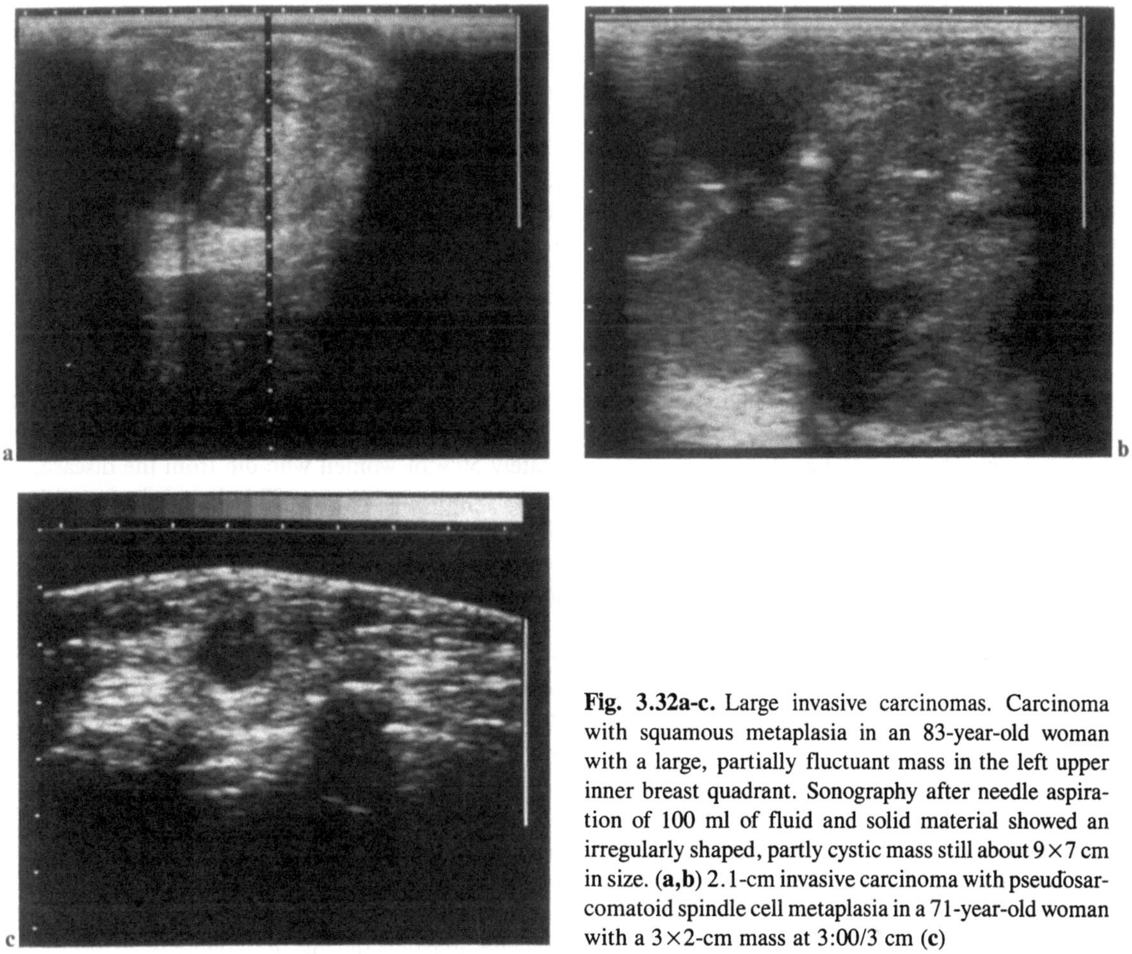

Fig. 3.32a-c. Large invasive carcinomas. Carcinoma with squamous metaplasia in an 83-year-old woman with a large, partially fluctuant mass in the left upper inner breast quadrant. Sonography after needle aspiration of 100 ml of fluid and solid material showed an irregularly shaped, partly cystic mass still about 9×7 cm in size. (**a,b**) 2.1-cm invasive carcinoma with pseudosarcomatoid spindle cell metaplasia in a 71-year-old woman with a 3×2-cm mass at 3:00/3 cm (**c**)

Metastasis of Breast Carcinoma

The site most frequently involved by metastasis from breast carcinoma is the ipsilateral axillary lymph nodes. While Haagensen (1971) stated that the frequency of axillary lymph node metastasis depends directly on the size of the primary tumor, reaching about 40% in a series of 922 cases, Hellman and colleagues (1982) reported a 74% frequency of axillary metastasis in autopsies of 303 women with breast carcinoma.

Palpable axillary lymph nodes usually can be readily demonstrated with ultrasound. Even with a relatively small primary tumor, large axillary metastases may have developed (Figs. 3.33, 3.34). With the immersion method, it is sometimes possible to document the primary tumor and axillary metastases on one image. But a hand-held real-time scanner is equally capable of documenting both lesions by the simple juxtaposition of scans (Fig. 3.35). In primary as well as follow-up examinations, ultrasound can help to delineate palpable axillary masses and guide their evaluation by needle biopsy (Fig. 3.36).

Axillary metastases of breast carcinoma appear on sonograms as faintly or softly marginated, hypoechoic foci, usually with regular, homogeneous internal echoes and no secondary phenomena. It is questionable whether the ability to demonstrate axillary lymph nodes with ultrasound in a patient with breast carcinoma is always indicative of metastasis, because lymph nodes enlarged by inflammation also can be visualized with ultrasound (Fig. 3.37). Axillary abscesses, moreover, may be indistinguishable from lymph nodes both clinically and sonographically (Fig. 3.38).

Besides axillary node metastases, sonography can disclose intramammary metastases and recurrent carcinomas in mastectomized areas or in residual tissue following prosthetic replacement (Figs. 3.39–3.41).

An important application of ultrasound in the setting of breast carcinoma is hepatic sonography to evaluate for distant metastasis. The liver ranks third in frequency (after the lung and bones) as a site for distant metastasis from breast carcinoma. Bässler (1978) reported that appxoximately 48% of all women with breast carcinoma, and approximately 59% of women who die from the disease, have hepatic metastases. This is consistent with the results of Hellman and colleagues (1982), who found a 60% incidence of hepatic metastasis in autopsies of 303 women with breast cancer.

Table 3.5. Relationship of hypoechoic to hyperechoic hepatic metastases from breast carcinoma.

Study	Metastases: Hypoechoic (*n* of cases)			Metastases: Hyperechoic (*n* of cases)	
Delmore and Hammer, 1982	31		:	4	
Weiss and Weiss, 1983	21		:	3	
Schölmerich et al., 1984	38		:	11	
Székessy et al., 1985	24		:	7	
Our results	16		:	2	
Total	130	(83%)	:	27	(17%)

Hepatic metastases of breast carcinoma may appear hypoechoic or hyperechoic on sonograms, with the hypoechoic pattern predominating (Table 3.5, Figs. 3.42b, 3.45). The causes of this behavior are not yet understood. Hepatic metastases have been seen to change from hypoechoic or hyperechoic and vice versa, and occasionally this has been observed in connection with systemic therapies. In two of our patients with initially hypoechoic hepatic metastases, hyperechoic lesions became apparent during the course of cytostatic therapy (Fig. 3.47).

An hepatic lesion detected with ultrasound in a patient with breast carcinoma can be difficult to identify as metastasic. Hepatic metastasis can be simulated by anatomic features such as the caudate lobe, quadrate lobe, or Riedel's lobe (Fig. 3.43) as well as by cysts (Fig. 3.44), hematomas, adenomas, primary hepatocellular carcinomas, hemangiomas (Fig. 3.46), and the lesions of focal nodular hyperplasia.

Diffuse hepatic metastasis has very marked and characteristic sonographic features, consisting of multiple hypoechoic foci that are partly discrete and partly coalescent (Figs. 3.48, 3.49).

It is possible for carcinomas of other organs to metastasize to the breast or, like primary breast carcinoma, to metastasize to the axillary or supraclavicular nodes (Figs. 3.50–3.52).

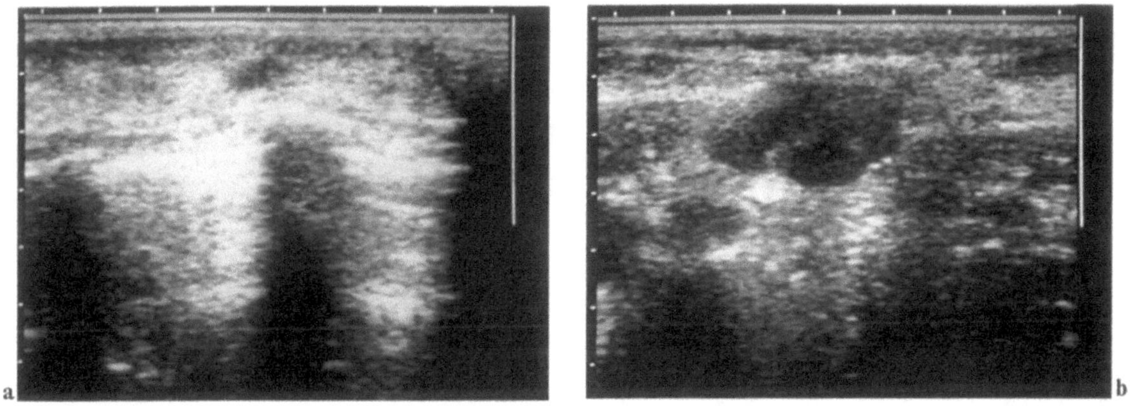

Fig. 3.33a,b. 5-mm simple solid carcinoma (**a**) with axillary lymph node metastases (**b**) in a 49-year-old woman with bloody nipple discharge, a pea-size mass in the right breast lateral to the nipple, and enlarged axillary lymph nodes

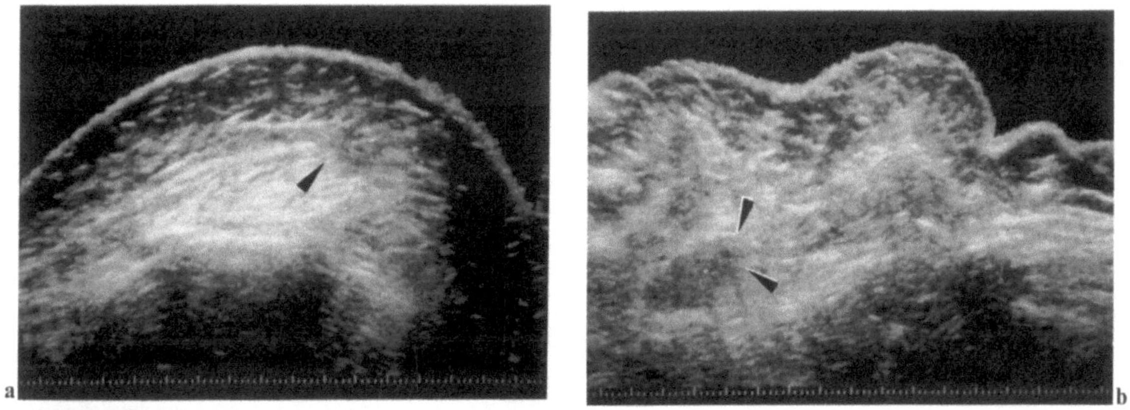

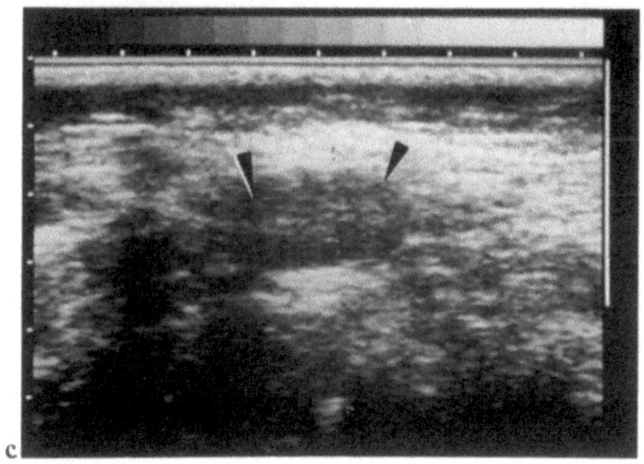

Fig. 3.34a-c. 1.6-mm infiltrating solid-cribriform carcinoma (**a**) with a large axillary metastasis (**b,c**) in a 46-year-old woman with a 2-cm mass at 12:00/4.5 cm in the left breast and palpable axillary nodes

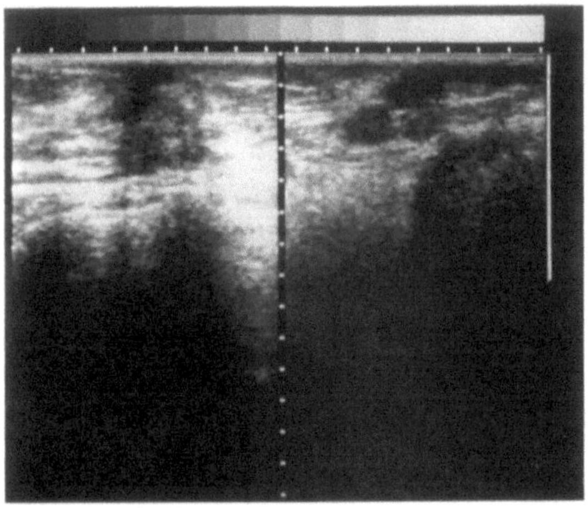

Fig. 3.35. Large infiltrating breast carcinoma (left) with axillary metastasis (right) documented on one image

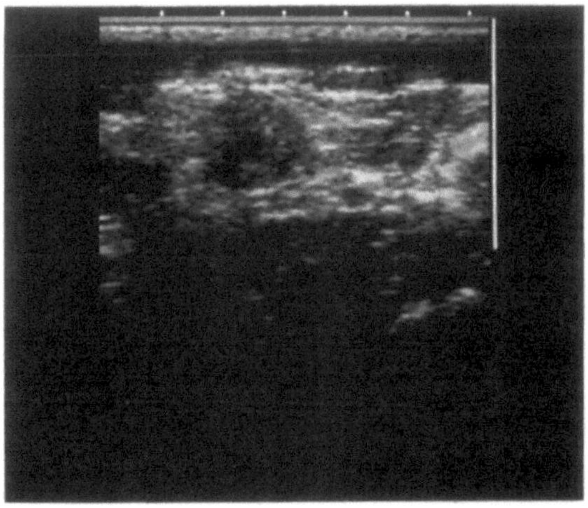

Fig. 3.36. Axillary metastasis of breast carcinoma in a 27-year-old woman who underwent mastectomy 9 months previously

a

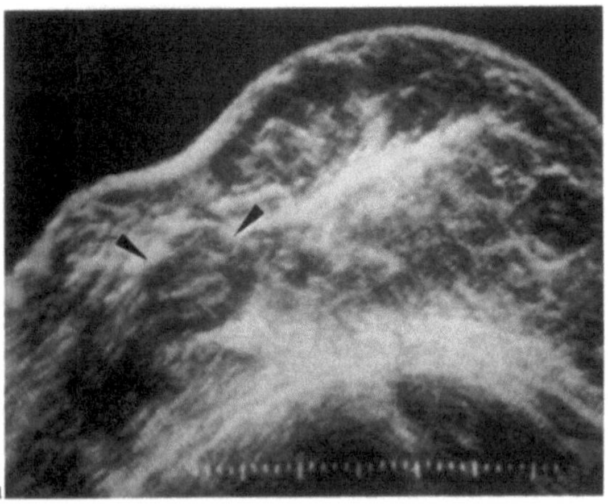

b

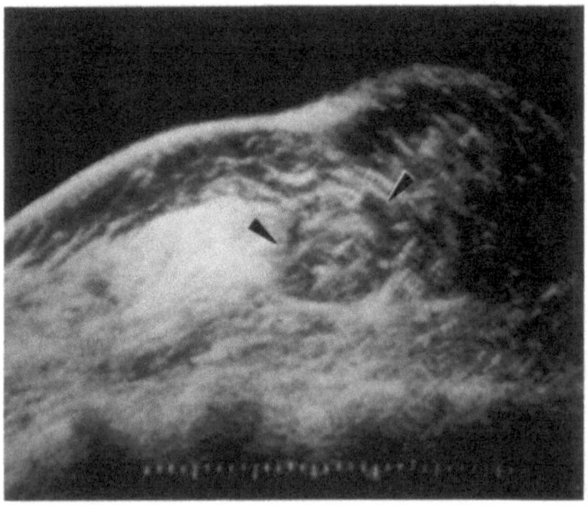

Fig. 3.37a,b. Calcified axillary lymph node 40 years after resolution of mastitis

a

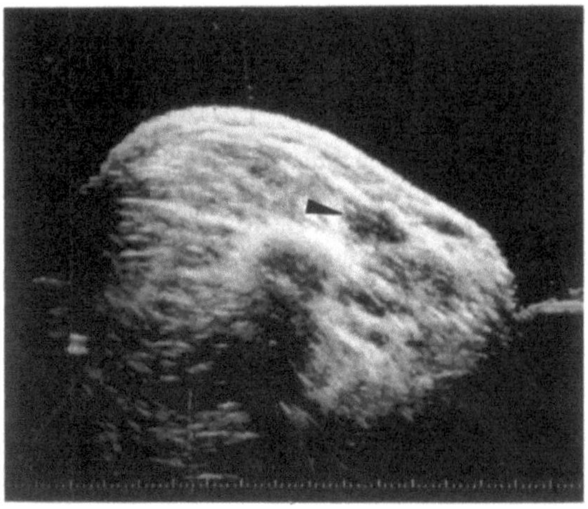

b

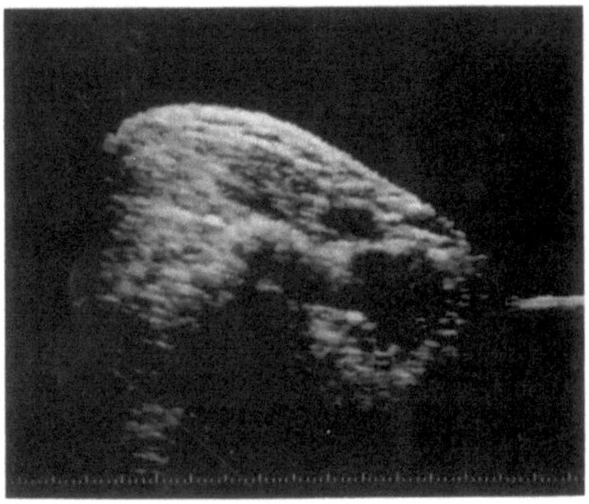

Fig. 3.38a,b. Cherry-size axillary mass in a 49-year-old woman with a normal-appearing ipsilateral breast. Fine-needle biopsy for suspected lymph node metastasis disclosed a purulent abscess that did not involve the nodes

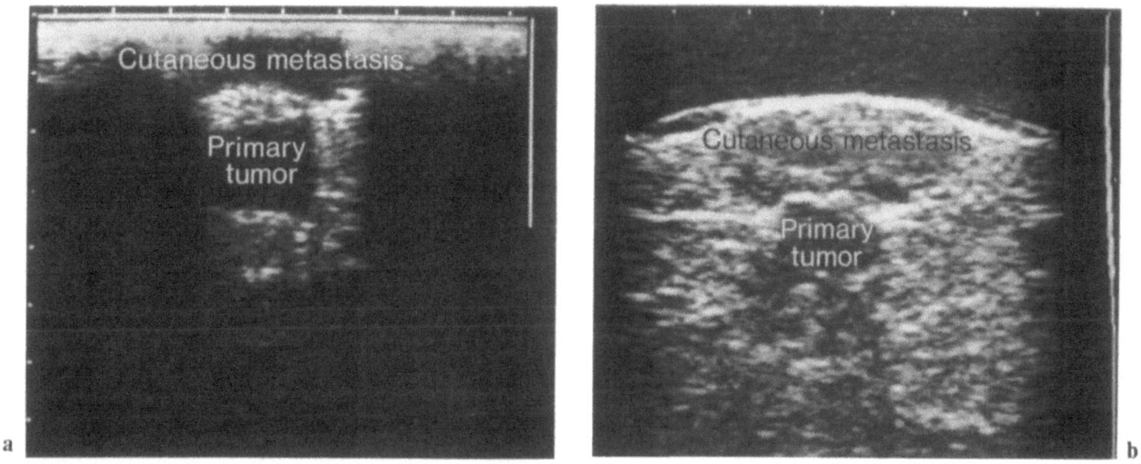

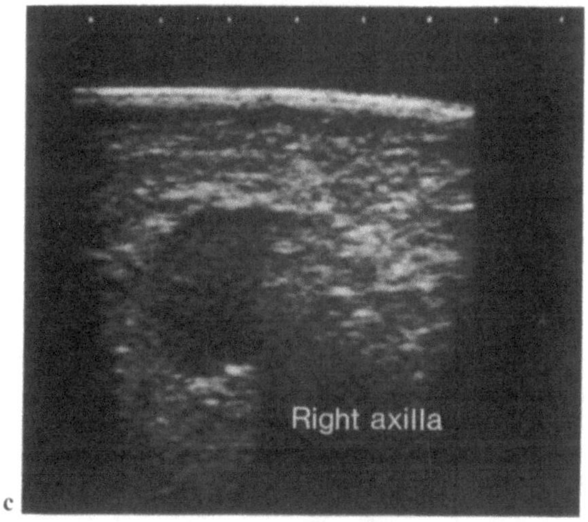

Fig. 3.39a-c. Cutaneous metastasis from a large infiltrating carcinoma in the right breast of a 65-year-old woman who also had axillary metastases

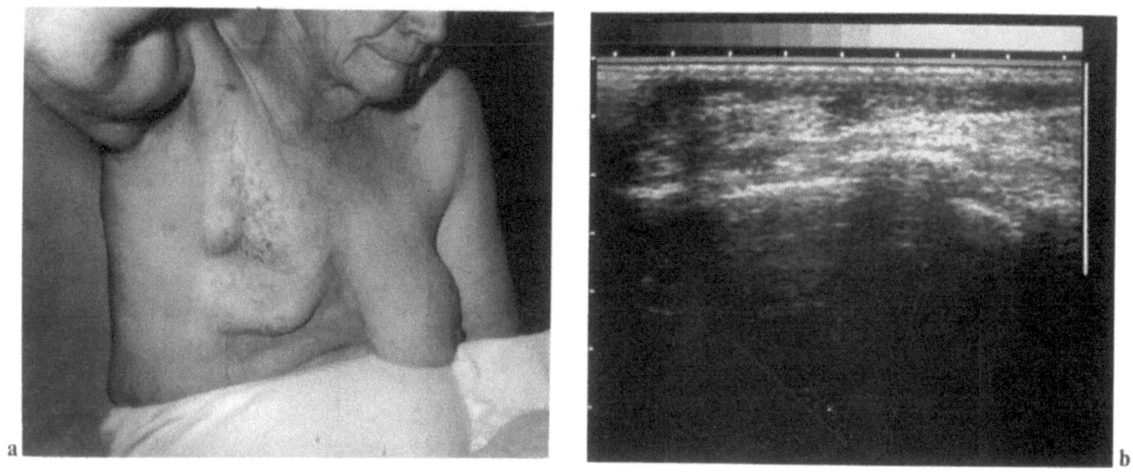

Fig. 3.40a,b. 5-mm local recurrence of breast carcinoma in a 79-year-old woman 13 years after mastectomy and radiation

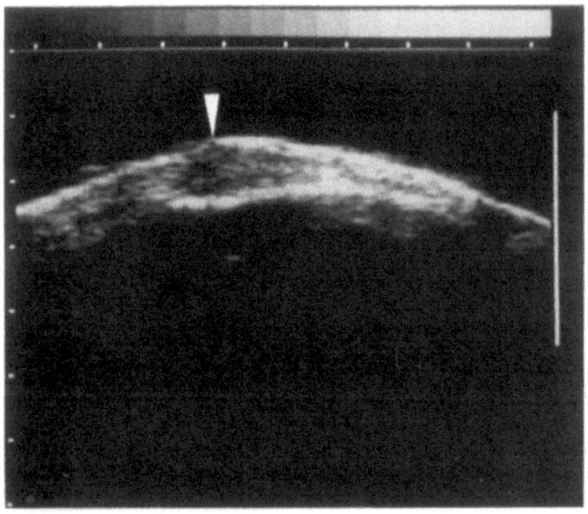

Fig. 3.41. Local recurrence of breast carcinoma in a 35-year-old woman 2 years after subcutaneous mastectomy, radiation, and prosthetic implantation

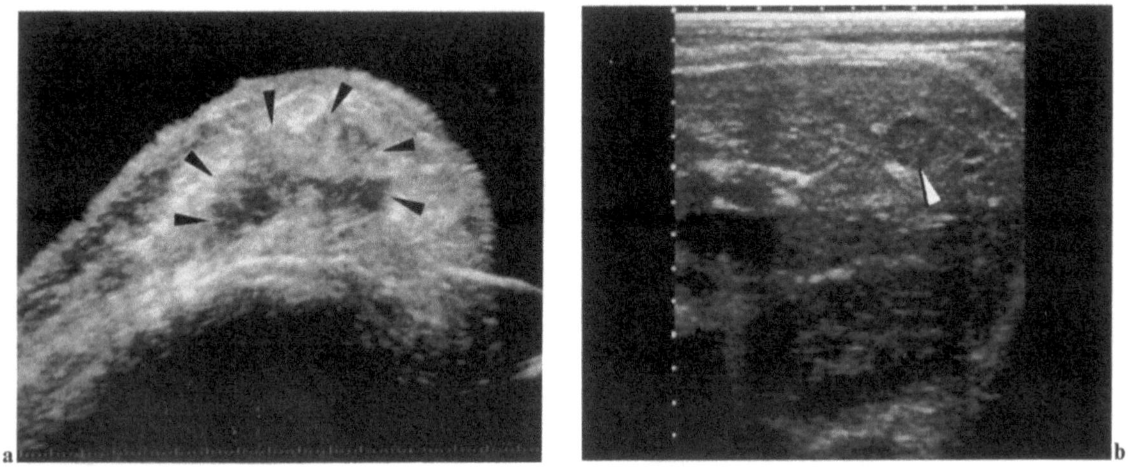

Fig. 3.42a,b. Large multicentric carcinoma (**a**) in the right breast of a 52-year-old woman with axillary metastases at the time of initial diagnosis. Hypoechoic hepatic metastases were detected about 1 year later (**b**)

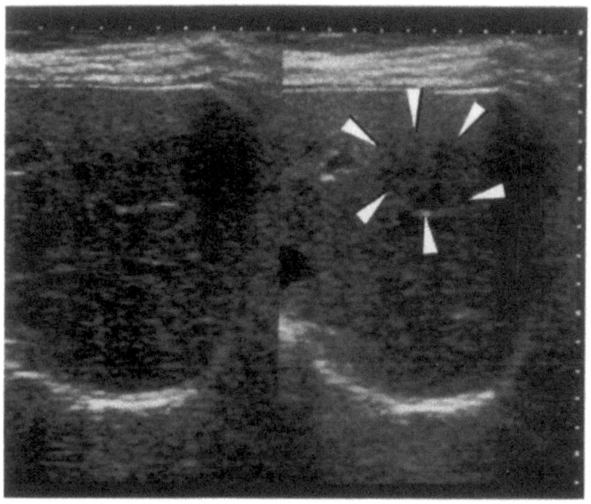

Fig. 3.43. Rounded, isoechoic to weakly hypoechoic mass in the liver of a 34-year-old woman with a 2.6-cm scirrhous breast carcinoma and axillary metastasis. Scintigraphy identified the mass as Riedel's lobe of the liver.

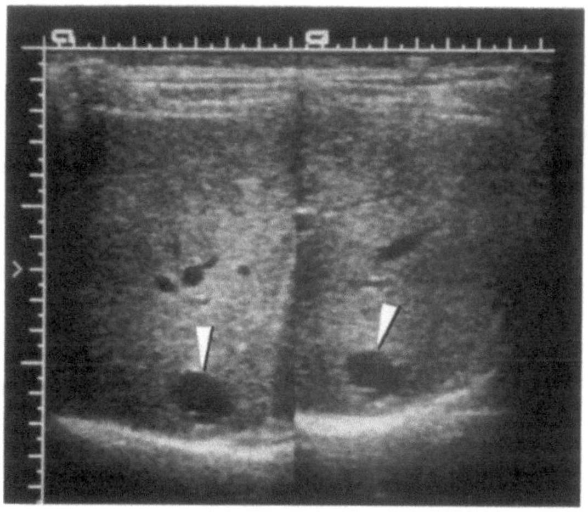

Fig. 3.44. Rounded, hypoechoic to anechoic mass in the liver of a 48-year-old woman with a 1.2-cm infiltrating scirrhous carcinoma and a 3-mm axillary micrometastasis. The mass was an hepatic cyst

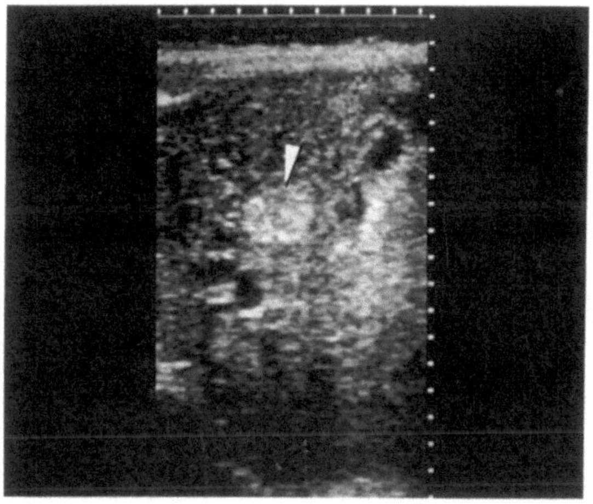

Fig. 3.45. Hyperechoic hepatic metatasis 21 months after mastectomy in 54-year-old woman who had a multicentric, invasive lobular breast carcinoma with eight confirmed axillary metastases at the time of operation

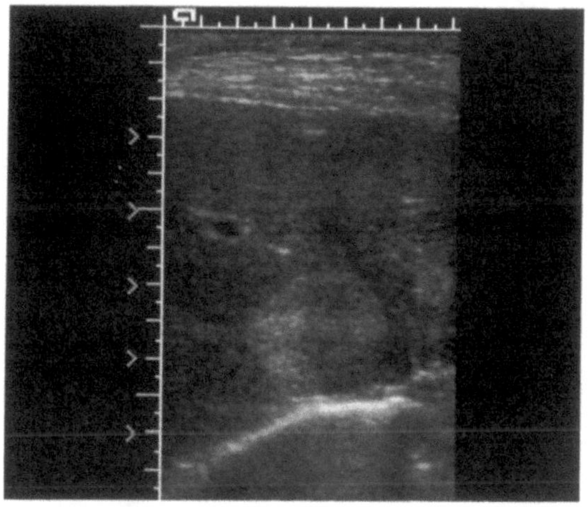

Fig. 3.46. Rounded, hypoechoic mass in the liver of a woman with a 1.5-cm simple solid carcinoma and three confirmed axillary metastases. Needle biopsy disclosed a cavernous hemangioma of the liver

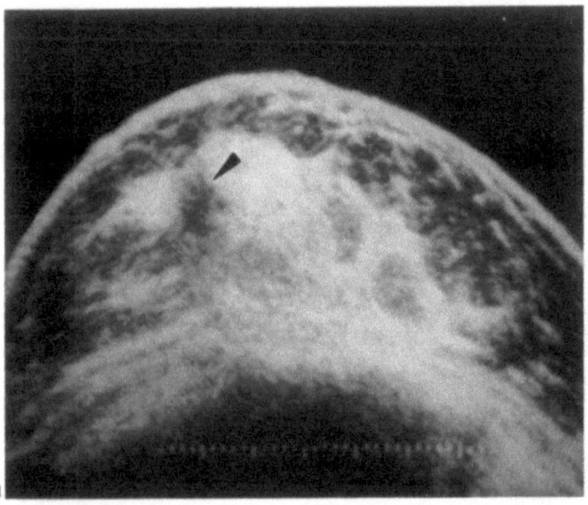
a

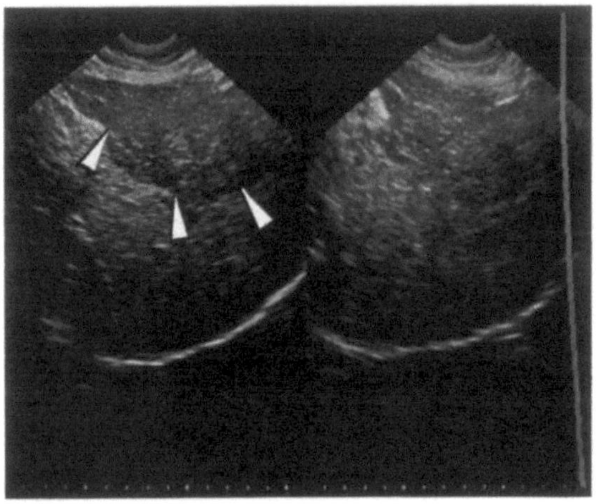
b

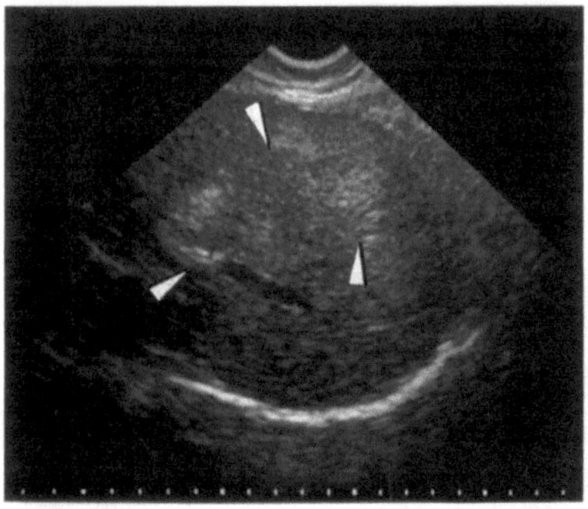
c

Fig. 3.47a-c. 3.2-cm simple solid carcinoma (**a**) in the left breast of a 48-year-old woman. Two axillary metastases were found at operation. About 4 years after mastectomy, ultrasound demonstrated a large hypoechoic mass in the liver (**b**) that was shown by excisional biopsy to be metastatic to the breast cancer. About 3 months later, after three cycles of adriamycin and cyclophosphamide, ultrasound showed hyperechoic foci in the liver with no further evidence of the hypoechoic mass (**c**)

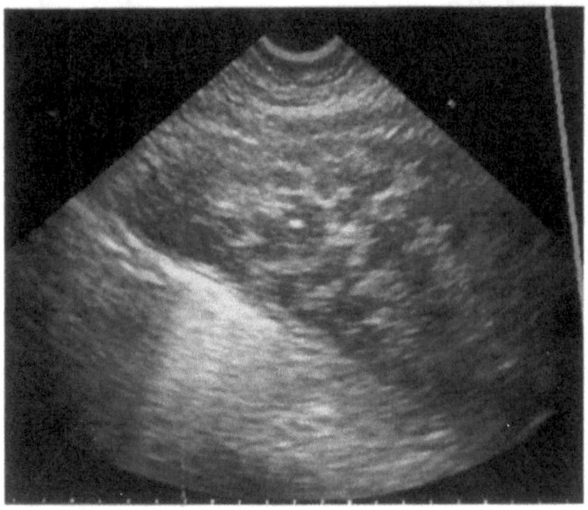

Fig. 3.48. Diffuse hepatic metastasis: **a** In a 41-year-old woman about 1 year after left mastectomy for a 21-cm scirrhous carcinoma with confirmed axillary micrometastasis

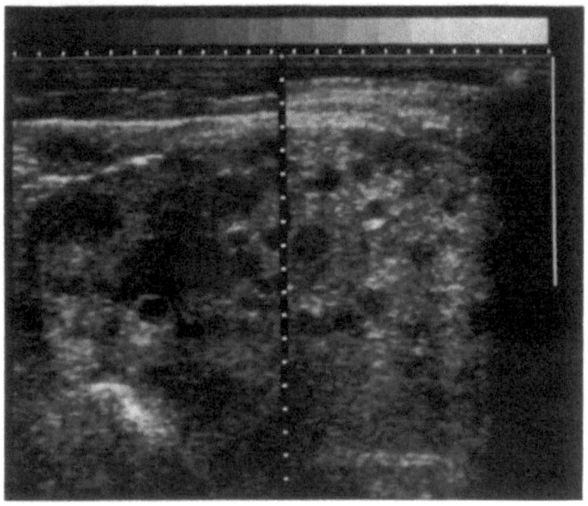

Fig. 3.49. Diffuse hepatic metastasis in a 48-year-old woman about 2 years after right mastectomy

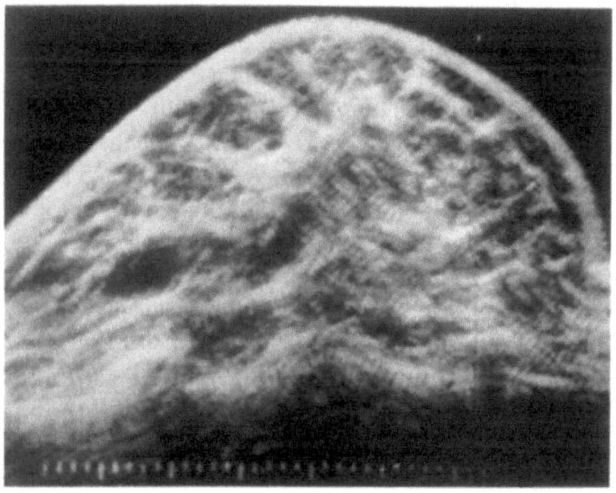

Fig. 3.50. 1.9-cm breast tumor metastatic to malignant melanoma in a 41-year-old woman

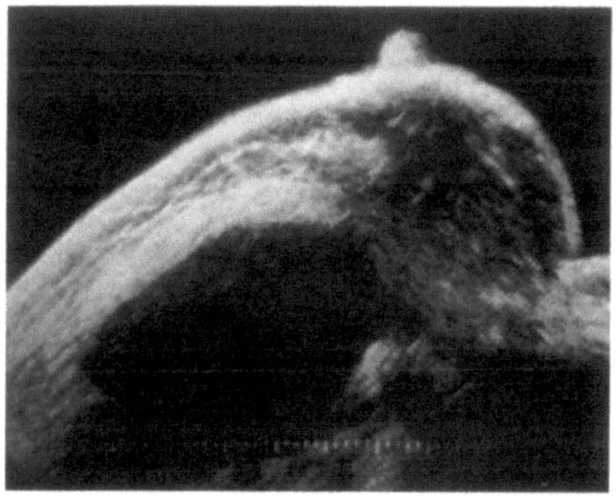

Fig. 3.51. Right breast of a 52-year-old woman has been invaded by a paraneoplastic process 11 years after the diagnosis of cervical carcinoma and 5 years after the detection of pulmonary deposits. Aspiration yielded 360 ml of a brown, opaque fluid found to contain malignant cells

a

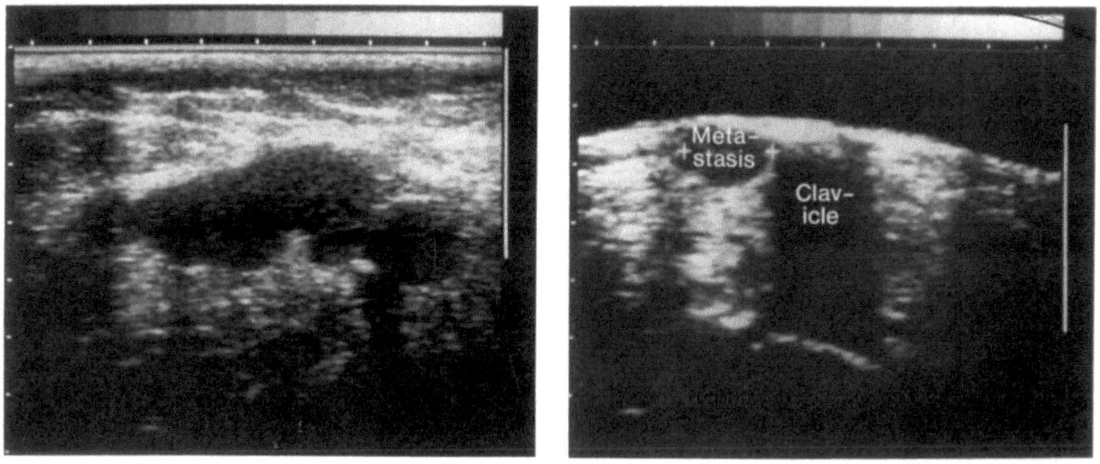

Fig. 3.52a,b. Axillary (a) and supraclavicular (b) metastases from ovarian carcinoma in a 64-year-old woman

Bibliography

Bässler, R. (1978). Pathologie der Brustdrüse. In Doerr, Seifert, Uehlinger (Eds.), *Spezielle pathologische Anatomie* (Vol. 11). Springer-Verlag, Berlin, Heidelberg, New York.

Becker, N., Frentzel-Beyme, R., Wagner, G. (1984). *Krebsatlas der Bundesrepublik Deutschland*. 2nd ed., Springer-Verlag, Berlin, Heidelberg, New York, Ch. 12, pp. 196–201.

Beeckman, P., Ampe, J., Berthot, J., Joe, G.T., Callens, B., Hoste, M. (1983). Echographic pattern of medullary breast carcinoma. *Journale Belge de Radiologie 66*:39–42.

Cole-Beuglet, C. (1982). Sonographic manifestations of malignant breast disease. *Seminars in Ultrasound 3*:51–57.

Cole-Beuglet, C., Soriano, R.Z., Kurtz, A.B., Goldberg, B.B. (1983). Ultrasound analysis of 104 primary breast carcinomas classified according to histopathologic type. *Radiology 147*:191–196.

Colin, C., Schaaps, J.P., Philippart, D. (1979). Interprétation des calcifications mammaires par l'echographie. *Annals of Radiology 22*:647–651.

Cooke, C.G., Grant, E.G., Cigaty, O.S. (1981). Ultrasound demonstration of giant malignant breast cyst undetected by xeromammography. *Journal of Clinical Ultrasound 9*:461–462.

Delmore, G., Hammer, B. (1982). Sonographische Hinweise auf den Primärtumor bei Lebermetastasen. In Kratochwil, Reinold (Eds.), *Ultraschalldiagnostik '81*. Thieme, Stuttgart, France, pp. 138–139.

Derchi, L.E., Rizzatto, G., Giuseppetti, G.M., Dini, G., Garaventa, A. (1985). Metastatic tumors in the breast: Sonographic findings. *Journal of Ultrasound in Medicine 4*:69–74.

Duda, V. (1982). *Ultraschall-Mammographie: Das sonographische Erscheinungsbild anatomischer und pathologischer Strukturen der Mamma unter Anwendung eines Immersionsscanners*. Dissertation, University of Marburg, West Germany, pp. 72–86.

Egan, R.L., McSweeney, M.B., Murphy, F.D. (1984). Breast sonography and the detection of cancer. *Recent Results in Cancer Research 90*:90–100.

Eulenburg, R, Lauth, G., Duda, V., Zwiens, G. (1984). Zur Differentialdiagnose des axillären Lymphknotens. *Röntgen-Blätter 37*:419–424.

Eulenburg, R., Lauth, G., Kalbfleisch, H. (1983). Seltene Malignome im Bereich der Mamma. *Geburtshilfe Frauenheilkunde 43*:387–391.

Grant, E.G., Holt, R.W., Chun, B., Richardson, J.D., Orson, L.W., Cigaty, O.S. (1983). Angiosarcoma of the breast: Sonographic, xeromammographic, and pathologic appearance. *American Journal of Roentgenology 141*:691–692.

Gros, Ch., Dale, G., Gairard, B. (1978). Breast echography: Criteria of malignancy and results. In Kurjak, A. (Ed.), *Recent Advances in Ultrasound Diagnosis. Excerpta Medica, Amsterdam-Oxford*, pp. 292–298.

Haagensen, C.D. (1971). *Diseases of the Breast*. 2nd ed. Saunders, Philadelphia, London, Toronto.

Hackelöer, B.J., Hüneke, B., Duda, V., Eulenburg, R., Laugh, G., Buchholz, R. (1981). Sonographische Differentialdiagnose der Mammakarzinome. *Ultraschall in der Medizin 2*:129–134.

Hackelöer, B.J., Lauth, G., Hüneke, B., Duda, V., Buchholz, R. (1981). Early detection of breast cancer: The value of ultrasound mammography. *British Journal of Radiology 54*:549–550.

Hellman, S., Harris, J.R., Canellos, G.P., Fisher, B. (1982). Cancer of the breast. In De Vita, Hellman, Rosenberg (Eds.), *Cancer: Principles and Practice of Oncology*. Lippincott, Philadelphia, Ch. 27.

Hiraide, H., Kawano, M., Hatsuse, K., Kadota, T., Kurokawa, T., Tamaki, K., Kanabe, S., Mizoguchi, O., Mimura, K., Iwasa, H. (1983). Case of breast cancer associated with Recklinghausen's disease. Gan No Rinsho. *Japanese Journal of Cancer Clincs 29*:1678–1681.

Igl, W., Lohe, K., Bassermann, R., Eiermann, W., Lissner, J. (1980). Früherkennung des Mamma-Carcinoms durch Ultraschall. Lecture, 1st World Congress on Senology, Hamburg.

Igl, W., Lohe, K., Kessler, M., Lissner, J. (1980). Mammacarcinom-Diagnostik mit Ultraschall. Lecture, German Congress on Roentgenology, Cologne.

Imamoto, H., Takatsuka, Y., Kawahara, T., Tokunaga, K., Morimoto, K. (1983). Ultrasonic diagnosis of early breast cancer. *Journal of the Japanese Society for Cancer Therapy 18*:1998–2003.

Jaworski, R.C., Kneale, K.L., Smith, R.C. (1983). Adenoid cystic carcinoma of the breast. *Postgraduate Medical Journal 59*:48–51.

Jellins, J., Kossoff, G., Reeve, T.S. (1975). Current and potential capabilities of ultrasound imaging for breast cancer diagnosis. *SPIE Medicine IV 70*:372–374.

Kasumi, F., Fukami, A., Kuno, K., Kajitani, T. (1982). Characteristic echographic features of circumscribed cancer. *Ultrasound in Medicine and Biology 8*:369–375.

Kelly-Fry, E., Sanghvi, N.T., Fry, F.J., Gardner, G., Gallager, H.S. (1978). Determination of alterations of phase angle of ultrasound transmitted through a malignant breast tumor. *Ultrasound in Medicine 4*:493–501.

Kobayashi, T. (1977). Gray scale echography for breast cancer. *Radiology 122*:207–214.

Kobayashi, T. (1978). Ultrasonic tissue characterization of breast cancer: Correlation of attenuation and echopattern. In Kurjak, A. (Ed.), *Recent Advances in Ultrasound Diagnosis*. Excerpta Medica, Amsterdam-Oxford, pp. 281–291.

Kobayashi, T. (1982). Ultrasonic detection of breast cancer. *Clinical Obstetrics and Gynecology 25*:409–423.

Kopans, D.B., Meyer, J.E., Proppe, K.H. (1981). The double line of skin thickening on sonograms of the breast. *Radiology 141*:485–487.

Kopans, D.B., Meyer, J.E., Steinbock, R.T. (1982). Breast cancer: The appearance as delineated by whole breast water path scanning. *Journal of Clinical Ultrasound 10*:313–322.

Kossoff, G. (1978). Ultraschall bei der Aufdeckung des Mamma-Frühcarcinoms. In *Brustkrebs-Früherkennung*. Fischer, Stuttgart, France, pp. 153–164.

Kossoff, G., Jellins, J., Reeve, T.S. (1978). Ultrasound in the detection of early breast cancer. *Cancer Campaign 1*:149–158.

Lauth, G., Duda, V., Eulenburg, R., Hackelöer, B.J., Hüneke, B. (1984). Möglichkeiten und Grenzen der Brustkrebs-Früherkennung mittels Ultraschallmammographie. *Röntgenpraxis 37*:62–65.

Maturo, V.G., Zusmer, N.R., Gilson, A.J., Bear, B. (1982). Ultrasonic appearance of mammary carcinoma with a dedicated whole-breast scanner. *Radiology 142*:713–718.

Mulz, D., Egger, H., Knüpfer, A., Althammer, G. (1981). Mikrokalk im Mammogramm und Darstellungsmöglichkeit im Ultraschall. *Geburtshilfe Frauenheilkunde 41*:255–258.

Nakano, A., Hamada, Y., Hirono, M., Hattori, T. (1982). Differentiation between pseudo- and malignant lymphoma of the breast—a case report. *Japanese Journal of Surgery 12*:76–78.

Reeve, T.S., Jellins, J., Kossoff, G., Barraclough, B. (1978). Ultrasonic visualization of breast cancer. *Australian and New Zealand Journal of Surgery 48*:278–281.

Reuter, K., D'Orsi, C.J., Reale, F. (1984). Intracystic carcinoma of the breast: The role of ultrasonography. *Radiology 153*:233–234.

Schölmerich, J., Volk, B.A., Neuner, C., Fröhlich, J., Gerok, W. (1984). Aussagefähigkeit der Sonographie bei Lebermetastasen. *Deutsche Medizinische Wochenschrift 109*:326–329.

Székessy, T., Claussen, C., Fiegler, W., Pochhammer, K.F., Feßler, B., Felix, R. (1985). Sonographische diagnostik bei soliden raumforderungen der Leber. *Ultraschalldiagnostik 84*:50–51.

Wagai, T., Tsutsumi, M. (1981). Echographic differentiation of histological structure in breast carcinoma. Excerpta Medica, Congress Series 553:369–373.

Weiss, H., Weiss, A. (1983). *Ultraschall-Atlas (internistische Ultraschalldiagnostik mit schnellen B-Bild-Geräten)*. Edition Medizin, pp. 116–117, 122–123.

4 Other Lesions

Effects of Iatrogenic Measures on Breast Sonograms

Hematomas

Hematoma formation is a frequent sequel to surgery or fine-needle aspirations of the breast. Although hematomas are usually easy to detect clinically, it is often difficult to establish their total extent. Ultrasound is the diagnostic study of choice in these cases. Fresh hematomas appear as predominantly cystic or anechoic masses with relatively ill-defined borders (Figs. 4.1, 4.2). Older, more organized hematomas present as solid masses, and diagnosis must be established by needle aspiration (Fig. 4.3).

Scars and Tissue Defects

Operative procedures on the breast produce scars and tissue defects that can be deceptively similar to carcinomas in their sonographic appearance. Areas of scar fibrosis can exhibit broom-straw-like projections as well as dense acoustic shadows (Figs. 4.4, 4.5), complicating the early detection of pathologic changes by sonography as well as by palpation and radiography. These diagnostic problems are not a cause for pessimism, but rather should motivate examiners to obtain clear sonographic documentation of corresponding cicatricial structures so that they will be able to recognize any changes that arise on follow-up examinations. Evaluation becomes extremely difficult in breasts with marked keloid formation (Fig. 4.6).

Mammoplastic Procedures

Mammoplastic operations radically alter the architecture of the breast tissue. In patients who have had reduction mammoplasty, the central region of the breast is very difficult to evaluate due to transplantation of the nipple-areolar pedicle and the presence of other scar tissue (Fig. 4.7).

Breasts that have had augmentation mammoplasty generally are easy to evaluate with ultrasound. Normally the implant will appear as a conspicuous anechoic structure with smooth borders. The area between the skin and implant is more clearly demonstrated by the immersion or water-bag method; to visualize the area behind the prosthesis, compression should be applied (Figs. 4.8, 4.9). Occasionally, peripheral scattered echoes are seen that may extend to the center of the prosthesis if the surface of the implant is wavy (Fig. 4.10). The cranial portions of a teardrop-shaped implant usually are difficult to evaluate on transverse scans – a problem that is easily solved by obtaining a longitudinal scan (Fig. 4.11). A capsular fibrosis diagnosed by palpation has its sonographic correlate in a thickened, often patchy-appearing prosthetic capsule (Fig. 4.12).

Mastectomy and Radiation to the Breast

Palpation has traditionally been the primary method for evaluating mastectomy scars, due to the limitations of X-ray mammography and thermography in this area. But sonography also can be a source of useful information. The normal mastectomy scar is easily evaluated with a short-focus transducer. A thin layer of fat and connective tissue is demonstrable between the skin and pectoral muscles (Fig. 4.13). Radiation leads to fibrosis of the skin and subcutaneous tissue, producing a marked rise of echogenicity (Fig. 4.14). This implies that it should be easy to detect hypoechoic tumor recurrences in such tissue. While individual cases support this assumption, we do not yet have conclusive evidence that sonography is of value in this area. Such a capability would be highly advantageous in following the growing number of breast cancer patients who are treated by local excision and subsequent radiation (Fig. 4.15).

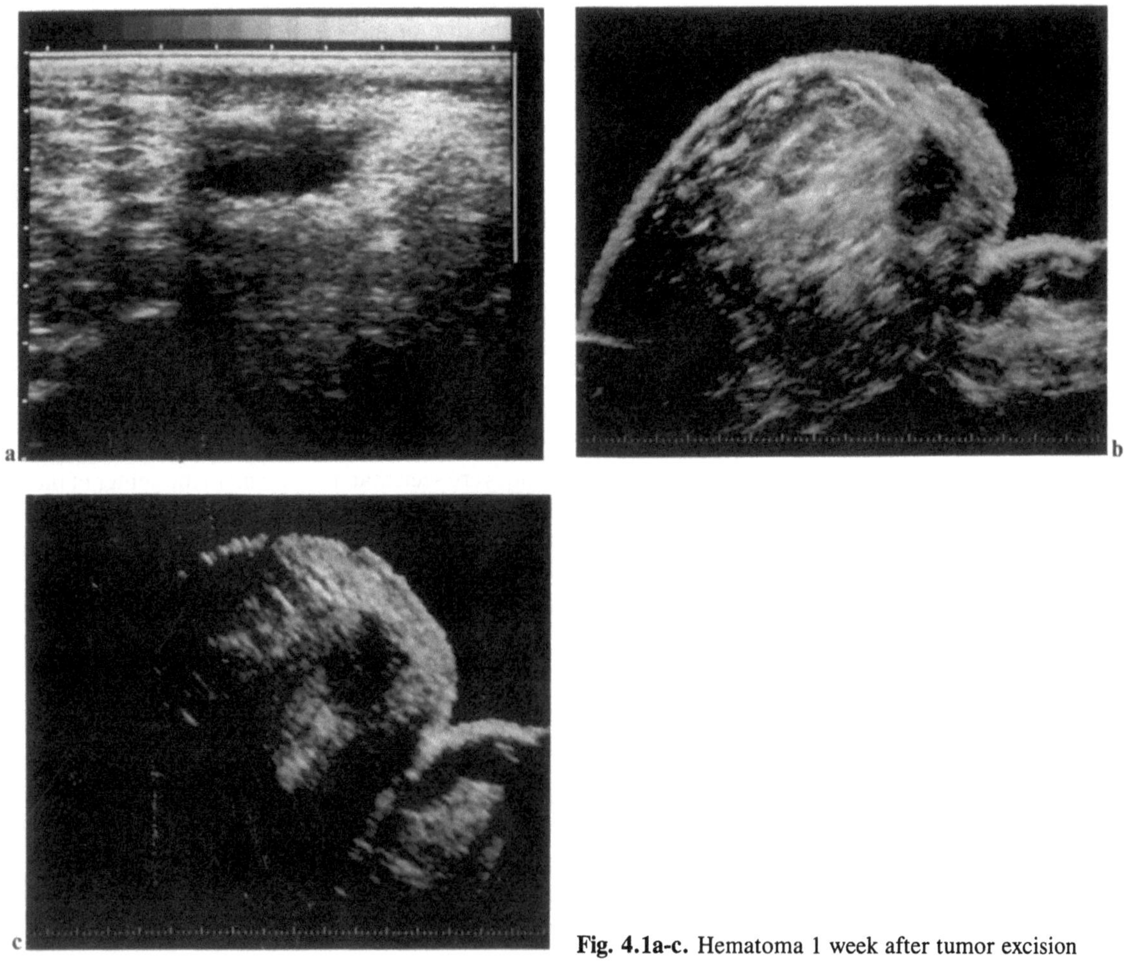

Fig. 4.1a-c. Hematoma 1 week after tumor excision

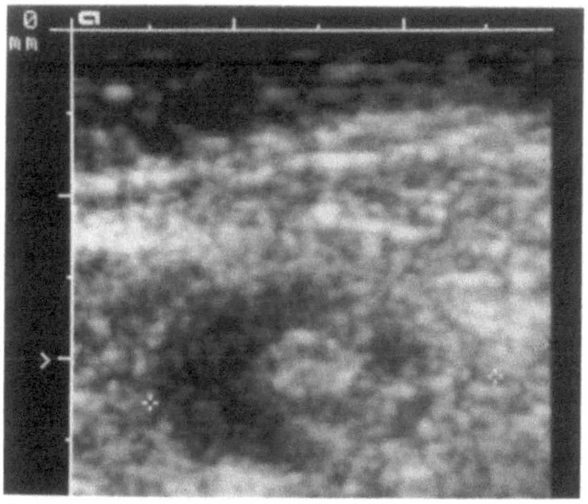

Fig. 4.2. Bleeding within a lymph node after fine-needle aspiration

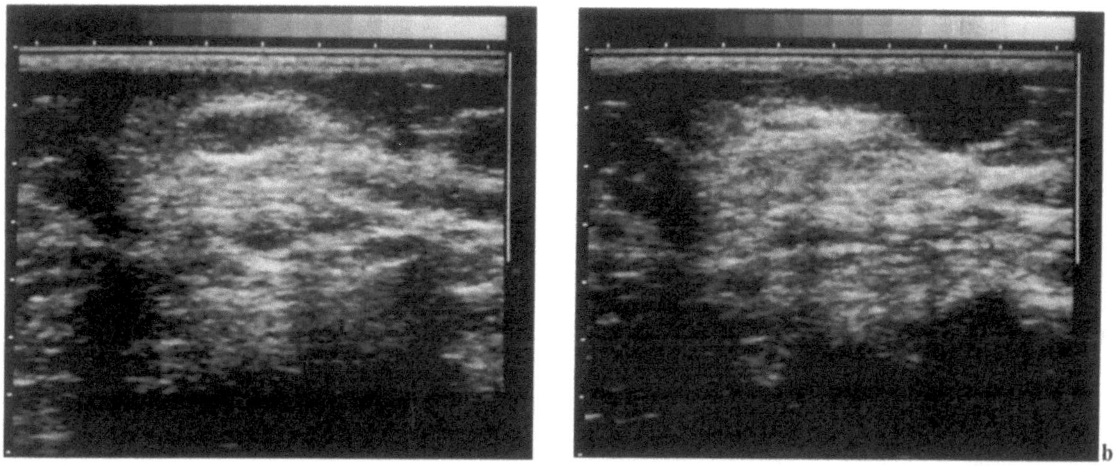

Fig. 4.3a,b. Solid mass discovered 1 week after fine-needle aspiration in that area (**a**). Repeat aspiration yielded blood, and the mass was no longer visible (**b**)

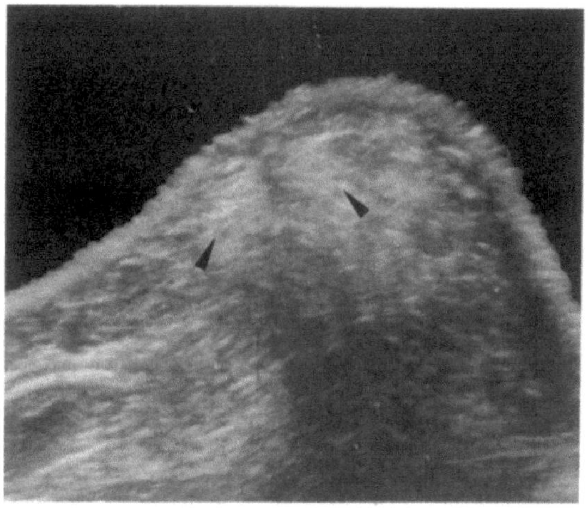

Fig. 4.4. Scar tissue 2 years after tumor excision, with architectural distortion and radial projections

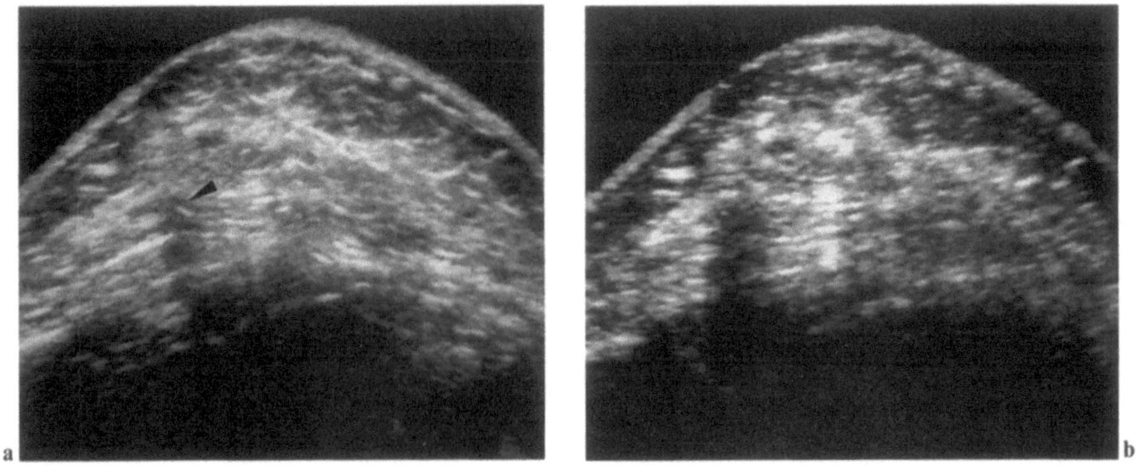

Fig. 4.5. Scar tissue producing a poorly marginated, hypoechoic lesion with radial projections and acoustic shadowing 16 years after tumor excision

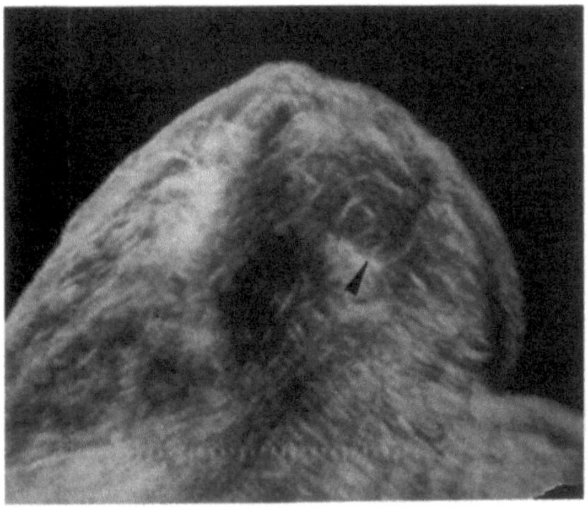

Fig. 4.6. Massive keloid formation in a 45-year-old woman about 20 years after multiple incisions were made for puerperal mastitis

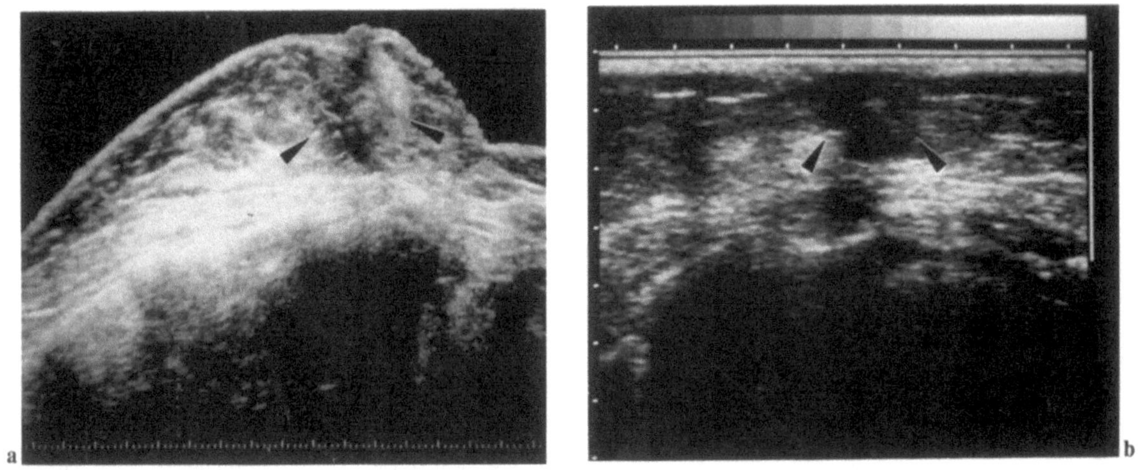

Fig. 4.7. Scans illustrating the extreme difficulty of evaluating the area of the "nipple pedicle" following reduction mammoplasty

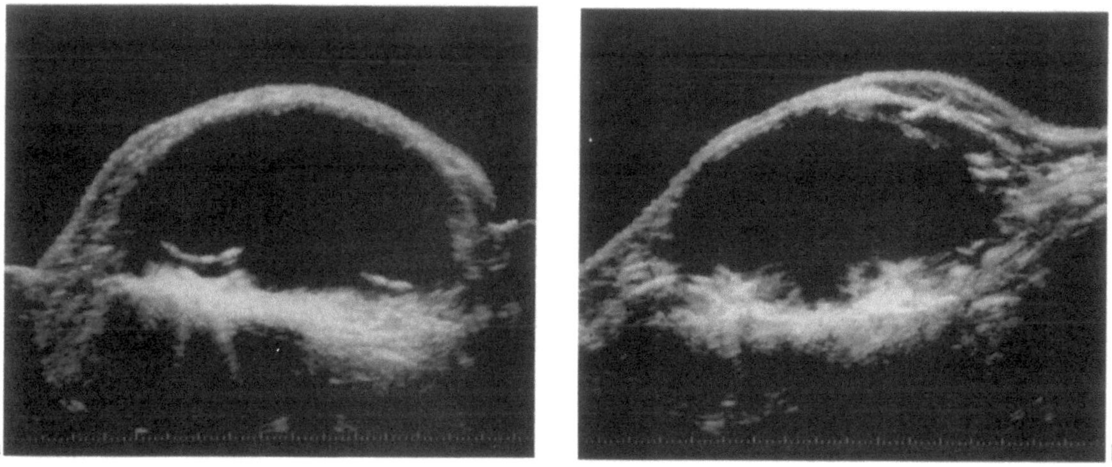

a b

Fig. 4.8a,b. Augmentation mammoplasty. **a** Inlay in place for about 1½ years

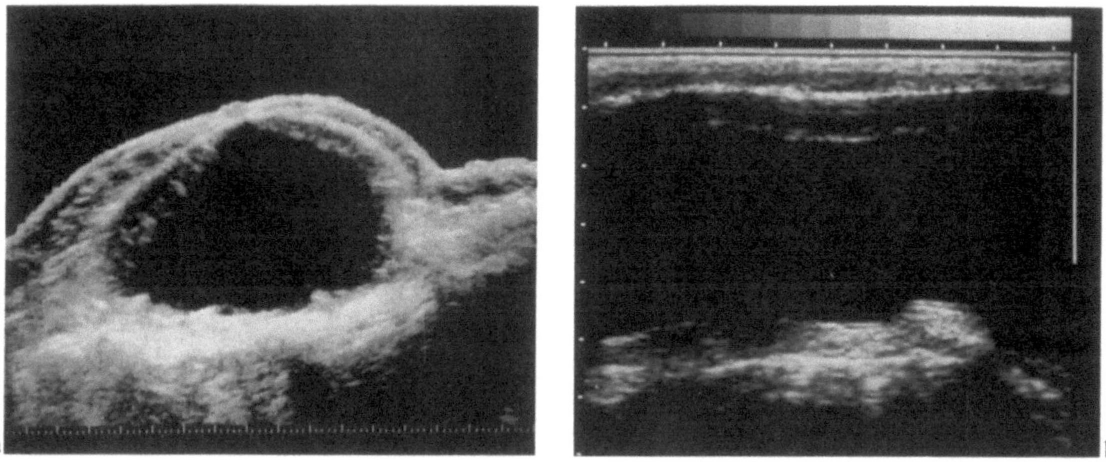

a b

Fig. 4.9a,b. Augmentation mammoplasty. Inlay in place for about 3 years

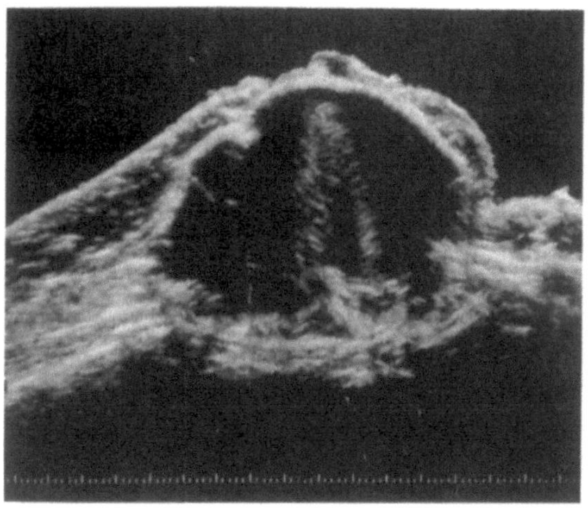

Fig. 4.10. Scattering echoes produced by the wavy surface of an 8-year-old prostheseis

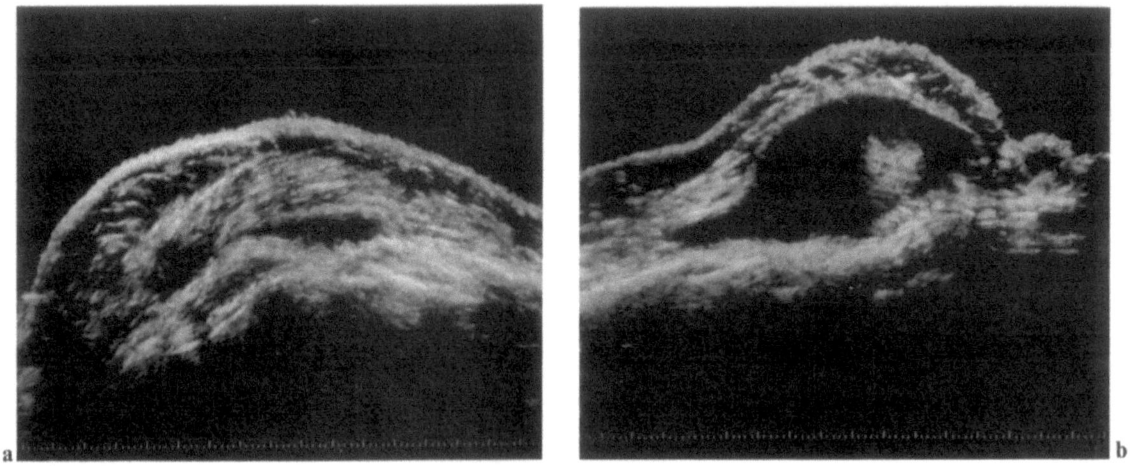

Fig. 4.11a,b. Teardrop-shaped breast prosthesis. The cranial portion is difficult to evaluate on the transverse scan (a) but is clearly visible on the longitudinal scan (b)

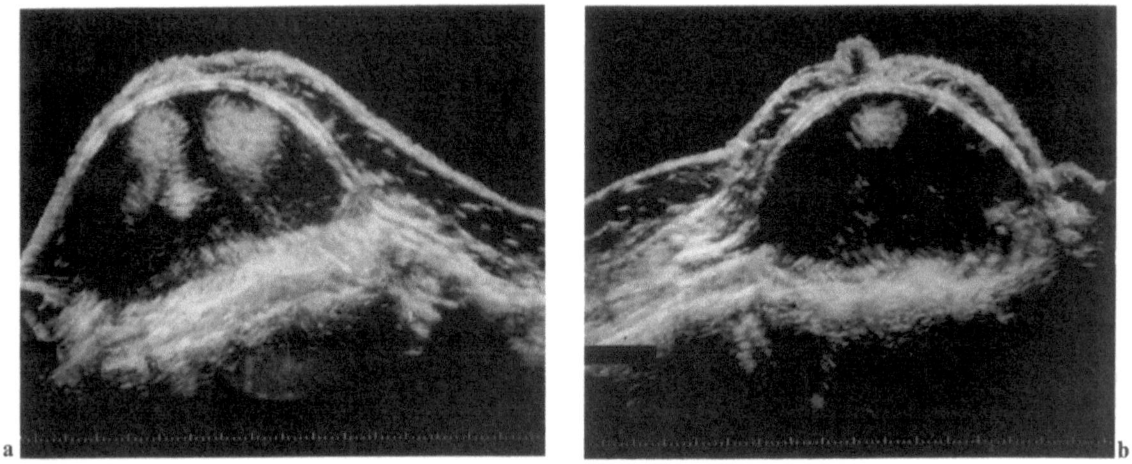

Fig. 4.12a,b. Capsular fibrosis. Thickened, patchy capsule of a prosthesis about 6 years old

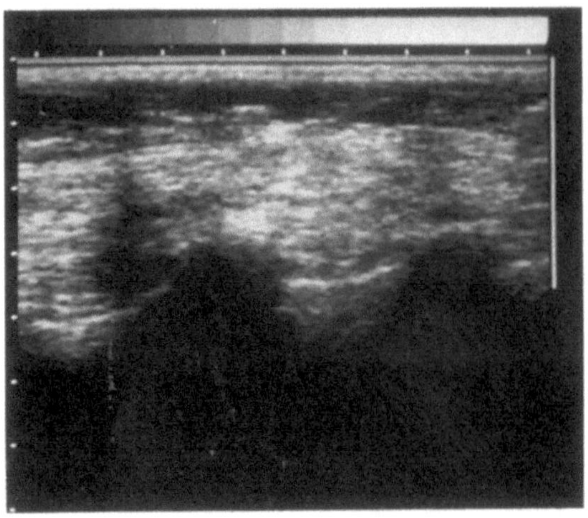

Fig. 4.13. Sonographic evaluation of mastectomy scar. Patient underwent mastectomy 7 years previously without radiation

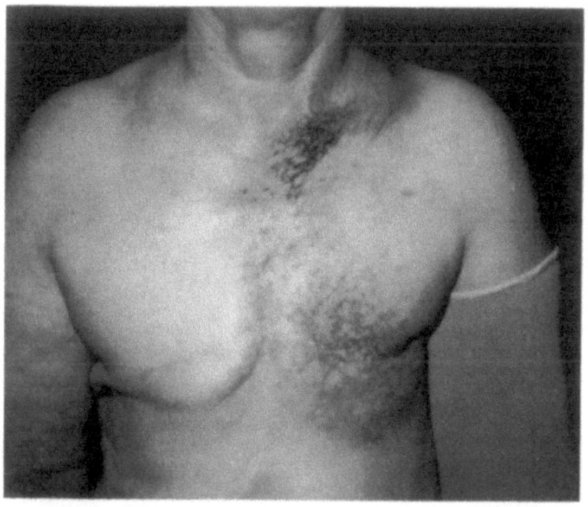

a

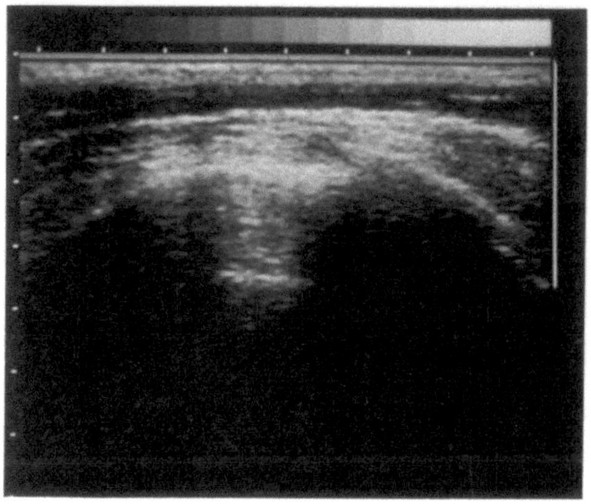

b

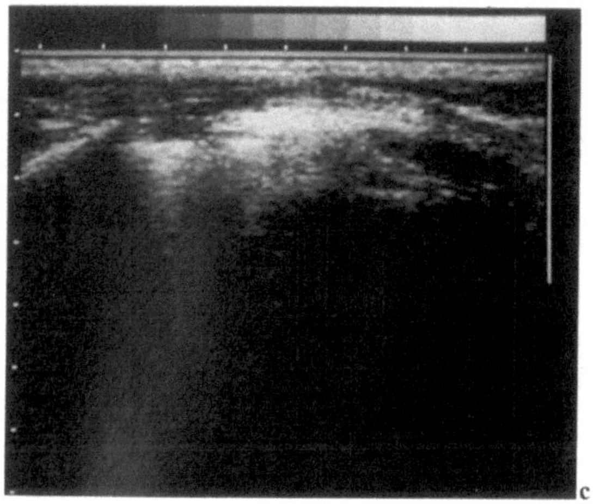

c

Fig. 4.14a-c. Bilateral mastectomy carried out 8 years previously with no radiation to the right side (**b**) and with postoperative radiation to the left side (**c**)

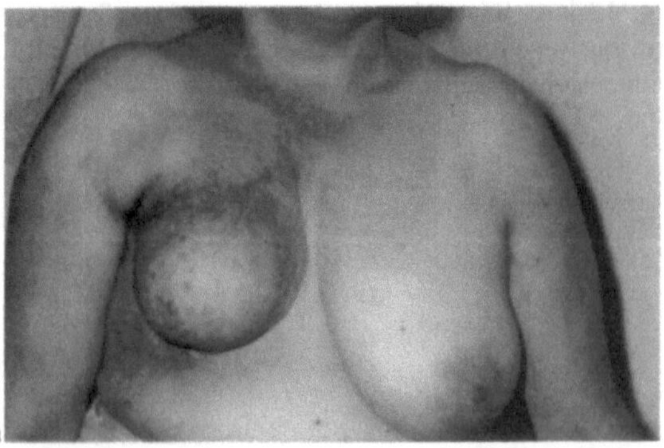

a

Fig. 4.15a-c. Patient treated 3 years previously by lumpectomy and radiation (**a,b**). The contralateral breast is shown for comparison (**c**)

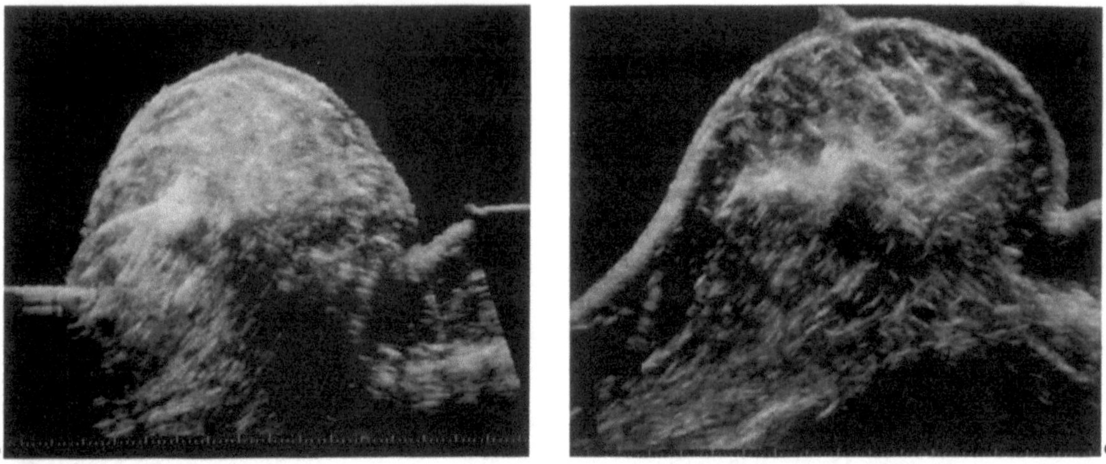

b

c

Gynecomastia

Gynecomastia in the pathologic sense refers to any hypertrophy of the male mammary gland or its rudiment. The sonographic pattern may be that of a small, homogeneous gland without a significant fat layer (focal type) or a larger, nonhomogeneous breast containing a substantial amount of fat (diffuse type). Both types may be hyperechoic throughout, or they may exhibit hypoechoic centers (Figs. 4.16, 4.17).

We distinguish the true gynecomastias (Fig. 4.18a) from neonatal gynecomastia caused by maternal hormones, pseudogynecomastia caused by fatty proliferation (Fig. 4.18), and neoplasms of the male breast. Although little sonographic experience is available with circumscribed tumors of the male breast, and especially with male breast carcinoma, such tumors do not appear to be essentially different from analogous lesions in the female breast (Fig. 4.19).

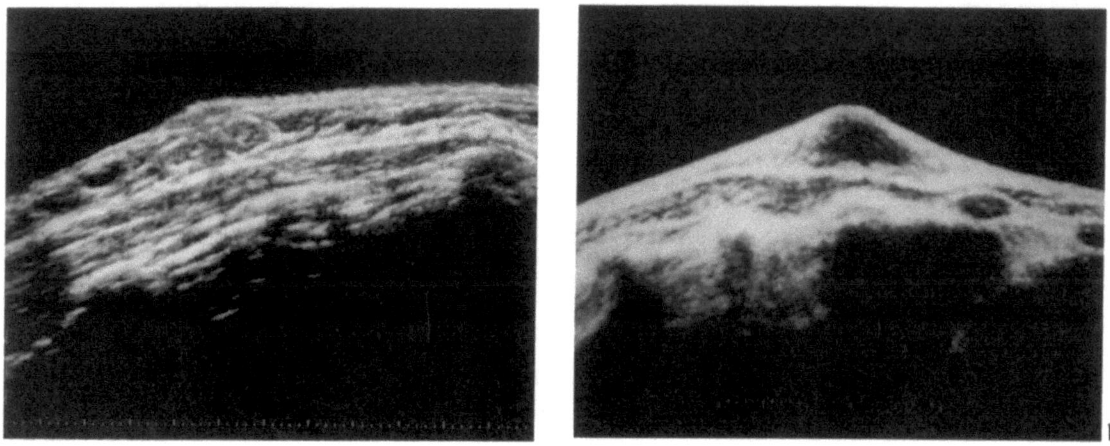

a b

Fig. 4.16a,b. Focal gynecomastia: hyperechoic type (**a**), hypoechoic type (**b**)

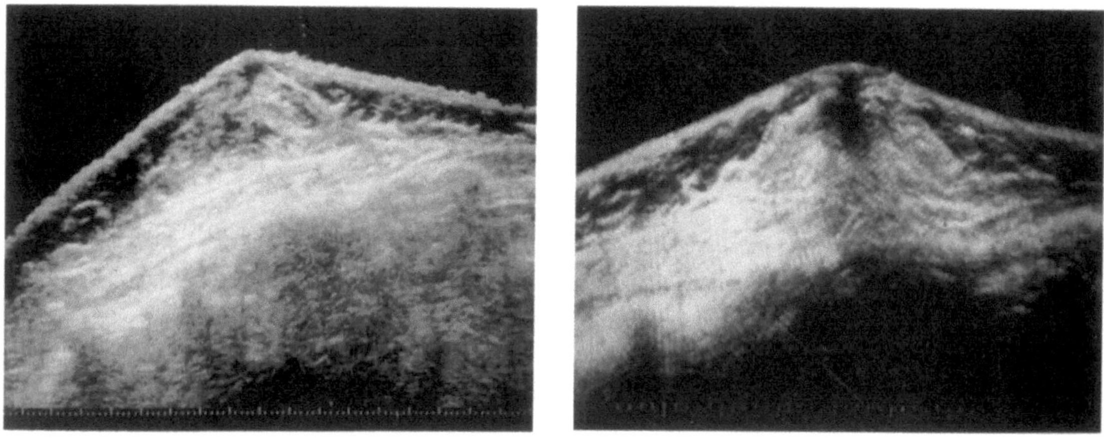

a b

Fig. 4.17a,b. Diffuse gynecomastia: hyperechoic type (**a**), hypoechoic type (**b**)

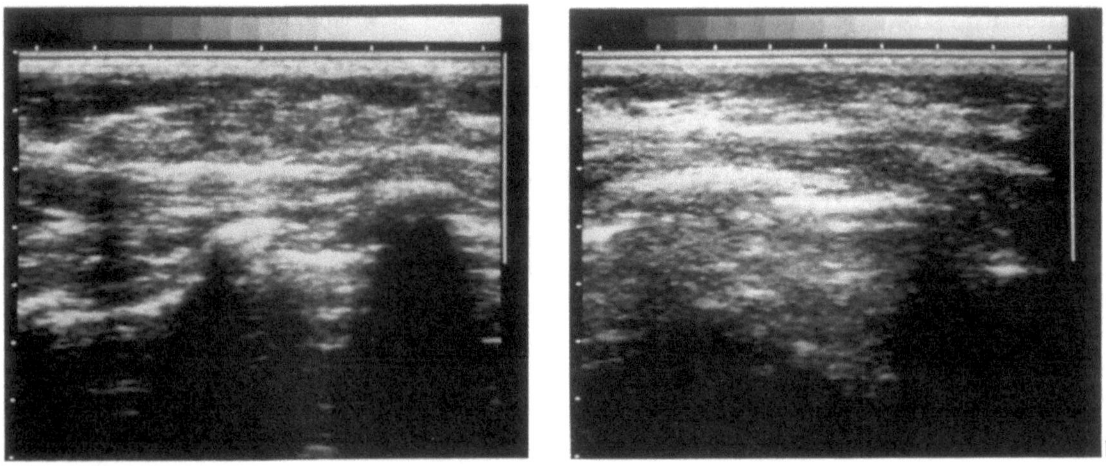

a b

Fig. 4.18a. "True" gynecomastia with glandular elements. **b** Pseudogynecomastia (fatty tissue only)

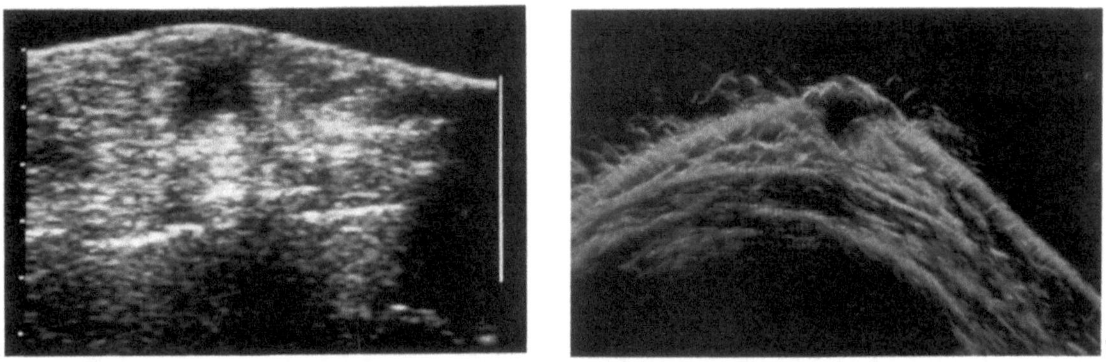

a b

Fig. 4.19a. Bloody nipple discharge and palpable mass in the left breast of man 59 years of age: breast carcinoma associated with gynecomastia. **b** Malignant lymphoma in the left breast of a 46-year-old male

Bibliography

Audretsch, W. (1975). Ultraschalldiagnostik bei Mammaprothesen nach operativer Behandlung von Mammatumoren oder Augmentationsplastik. *Geburtshilfe Frauenheilkunde 35*:853–858.

Cole-Beuglet, C., Schwartz, G.F., Kurtz, A.B., Patchefsky, A.S., Goldberg, B.B. (1982). Ultrasound mammography for male breast enlargement. *Journal of Ultrasound in Medicine 1*:301–305.

Cole-Beuglet, C., Schwartz, G., Kurtz, A.B., Patchefsky, A.S., Goldberg, B.B. (1983). Ultrasound mammography for the augmented breast. *Radiology 146*:737–742.

Duda, V. (1982). *Ultraschall-Mammographie: Das sonographische Erscheinungsbild anatomischer und pathologischer Strukturen der Mamma unter Anwendung eines Immersionsscanners*. Dissertation, University of Marburg, West Germany, pp. 94–97.

Eulenburg, R., Lauth, G., Duda, V. (1984). Gynecomastia and malignoma of the male breast. *Journal of Cancer Research and Clinical Oncology 107*, Suppl:20.

Grant, E.G., Richardson, E.D., Cigtay, O.S., Dritschilo, A., Lee, T.C. (1983). Sonography of the breast: Findings following conservative surgery and irradiation for early carcinoma. *Radiology 147*:535–539.

Jackson, V.P., Gilmor, R.L. (1983). Male breast carcinoma and gynecomastia: Comparison of mammography with sonography. *Radiology 149*:533–536.

Jellins, J., Kossoff, G., Reeve, T.S. (1975). The ultrasonic appearance of pathology in the male breast. *Ultrasound in Medicine and Biology 2*:43–44.

Meyer, J.E., Kopans, D.B. (1983). The appearance of the therapeutically irradiated breast on whole-breast water-path ultrasonography. *Journal of Ultrasound in Medicine 2*:211–213.

Rosenbaum, J.L., Bernardino, M.E., Thomas, J.L., Wigley, K.D. (1981). Ultrasonic findings in silicone-augmented breasts. *Southern Medical Journal 74*: 455–458.

Shafir, R., Heyman, Z., Tzur, H., Iztchak, Y. (1983). Ultrasound scanning as an aid in the diagnosis and treatment of periprosthetic hematoma after breast surgery. *Plasic and Reconstructive Surgery 71*:858–860.

Wigley, K.D., Thomas, J.L., Bernardino, M.L., Rosenbaum, I.L. (1981). Sonography of gynecomastia. *American Journal of Roentgenology 136*:927–930.

5
The Place of Sonography in Breast Diagnosis

Sonography Versus Palpation

In many cases it is possible to correlate a sonographically detected lesion with a clinically palpable mass. On the other hand, it is not unusual to find discrepancies between palpatory and sonographic findings. Thus, a tumor may be sonographically detectable but nonpalpable, or a palpable mass may not have a sonographic counterpart.

In lumpy breasts that appear to lack a subcutaneous fat layer, one can sometimes identify palpable masses as simple outpouchings of the glandular tissue with ultrasound (Fig. 5.1).

Islands of involution at the periphery of the mammary gland can mimic focal lesions on sonograms. Examination on the second plane will almost always disclose the true nature of this phenomenon (Fig. 5.2).

At this point we again caution examiners not to declare the presence of a focal lesion unless it can be demonstrated reproducibly on both planes.

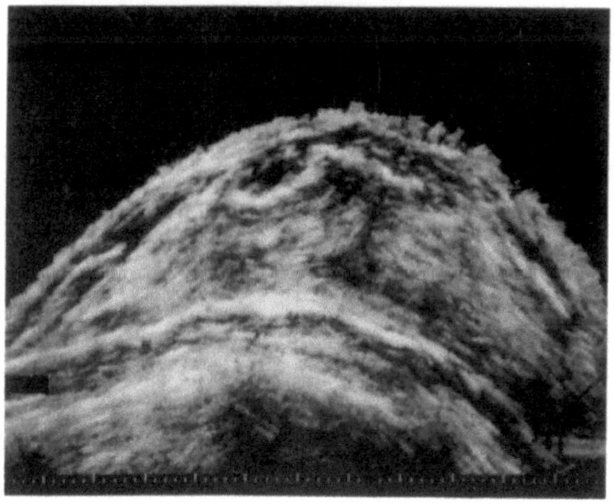

Fig. 5.1. Protrusions of glandular tissue in a 22-year old woman with a painful, lumpy breast

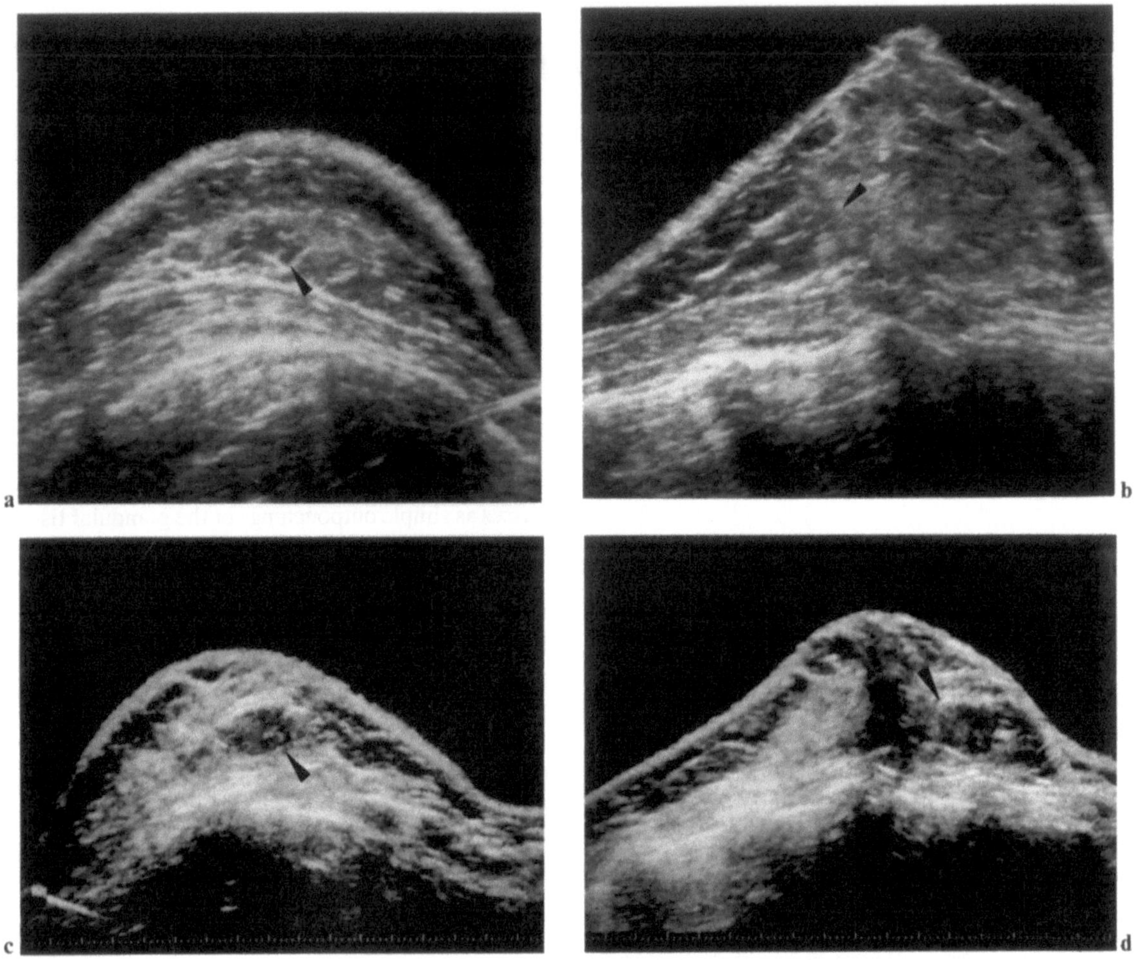

Fig. 5.2a,b. Fatty infiltration mimicking a focal lesion on the transverse scan (**a,b**). **c,d** Fibroadenoma whose internal structure resembles fat, but which is obviously a focal lesion when examined on both planes

Sonography Versus Thermography

Two main techniques of thermal imaging are presently available. One is telethermography (known also as infrared or electronic thermography), in which infrared radiation from the breast produces changes in the electrical resistance of a semiconductor crystal (indium antimonide or mercury cadmium telluride) cooled to the temperature of liquid nitrogen (=196°C). These resistance changes are used to construct an image. Amalric, Gautherie, and Gros in particular have helped to standardize the interpretation of the thermovascular patterns disclosed by this method (Amalric et al., 1972; Gautherie and Gros, 1980; Gautherie et al., 1984).

In liquid crystal thermography (called also contact or plate thermography), thermosensitive cholestric liquid crystals are deposited on thin films that are placed in contact with the skin to produce a colored "map" of the cutaneous heat pattern. Special emphasis is placed on the "dynamic" examination, in which the breast is cooled after initial thermography and then examined for the return of vascularity and for any blood vessels that appear to be resistant to cooling. Tricoire (1970, 1973) in particular has contributed much to standardizing the interpretation of liquid crystal thermograms.

In contrast to sonography and mammography, which portray morphologic substrates, thermography can accurately measure heat emission and thus provide information on the functional blood flow conditions within an organ. Abnormal patterns of vascularity and focal or global hyperthermia in the breast may be caused by tumors and inflammatory processes as well as by such factors as age, the phase in the menstrual cycle, general hormonal activity, pregnancy, and the use of oral contraceptives or other drugs. While tumors and inflammatory processes cause asymmetrical changes, the other factors tend to produce symmetrical patterns. Thermography is unable to distinguish between a neoplastic and an inflammatory cause of thermovascular change. If a suspicious thermogram is obtained, diagnosis can be aided by reexamining the patient in a different phase of the menstrual cycle, after antiinflammatory therapy, or after the discontinuation of vasoactive drugs or hormones. Atypical thermograms should always be an indication for further evaluation by mammography or sonography. Even if clinical, mammographic, and sonographic findings are negative, an abnormal thermogram should be considered a serious warning sign and should prompt the physician to schedule frequent follow-ups.

Fast-growing malignancies with increased metabolic activity lead to overheating of the blood. The overheated venous blood draining from the tumor causes increased thermal convection, which elicits thermographic changes on the skin surface. Owing to the ability of tumor cells to release vasoactive substances that raise the temperature of the overlying skin, even precancerous tumors and small, deeply situated carcinomas can produce abnormalities on thermal breast images. Thus, thermography can give evidence of malignant disease (especially when changes are progressive) several years before signs appear that would be detectable with other diagnostic methods. Particularly "hot" carcinomas usually have a short doubling time and thus imply a poor prognosis. They frequently represent stage III histologic grading and have a high association with axillary lymph node metastasis (Gautherie, 1983).

As stated above, thermography is incapable of distinguishing between hyperthermias caused by inflammatory and malignant processes. This is a

Table 5.1. Differential diagnosis of skin thickening in the breast.

Scar, keloid
Radiation
Mastitis
Inflammatory carcinoma
Cutaneous infiltration, ulceration
Cutaneous metastasis
Carcinomatous lymphangiosis
Lymphatic obstruction in the breast caused by
axillary metastases from breast carcinoma
axillary metastases from tumors of other organs
Hodgkin's and non-Hodgkin's lymphoma
elephantiasis (especially in women from the Indian subcontinent
mycosis fungoides
Upper inflow stasis caused by
mediastinal metastases
thrombosis (axillary vein, subclavian vein, vena cava)
right-sided heart failure ("unilateral" edems is possible!)
Anasaarca (cardiac, renal)
Leukemia
Tuberculosis
Scleroderma
Leiomyomatosis

Reprinted from Skaane et al., 1985, with permission.

particular problem in inflammatory carcinomas, which even clinically can closely resemble mastitides. Sonographically, both mastitis and inflammatory carcinoma are manifested by a mottling and thickening of the skin. In mastitis the skin contour usually appears to merge with the underlying tissue and cannot be clearly delineated from it. In carcinoma, on the other hand, the skin changes are often caused by carcinomatous lymphangiosis, in which the skin still appears mottled and thickened, but usually presents a double contour over its full extent. Differentiation becomes difficult in cases where the skin has been infiltrated by tumor. Moreover, skin changes in the breast can have a great variety of causes (Table 5.1; Skaane et al., 1985). The detection of abscess formation can aid in the diagnosis of mastitis, although the possibility of tumor necrosis should also be considered when an abscesslike mass is recognized. Thus, the differentiation of mastitis from inflammatory carcinoma can be difficult clinically, thermographically, and sonographically (Figs. 5.3, 5.4).

Fig. 5.3a-e. Nonpuerperal mastitis. Sonogram shows thickening and mottling of the skin with increased density of the subcutaneous fat layer

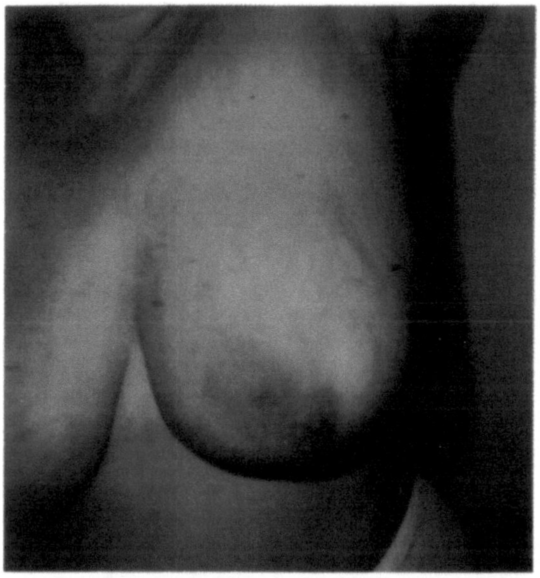

a

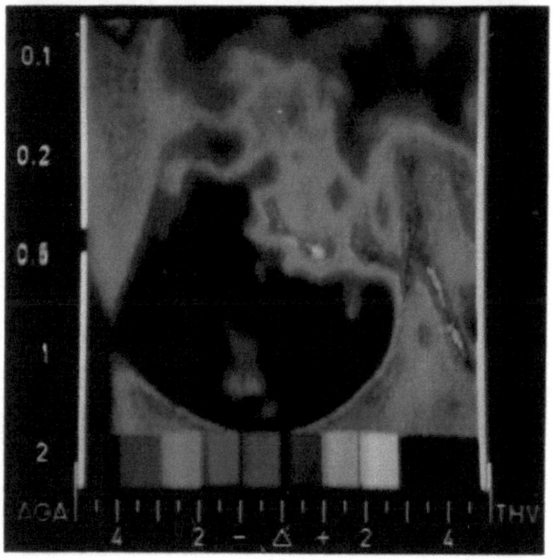

b

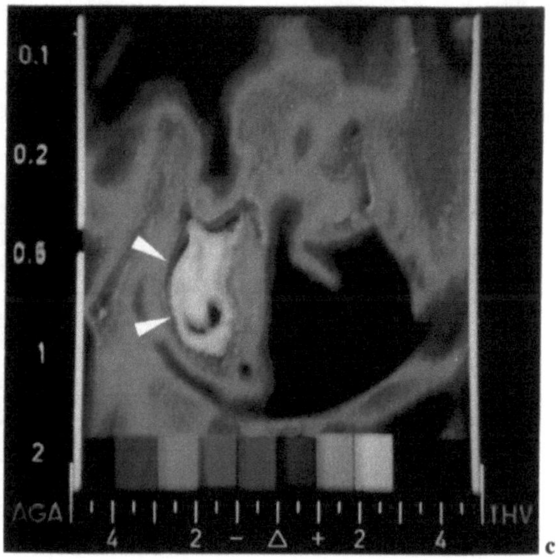

c

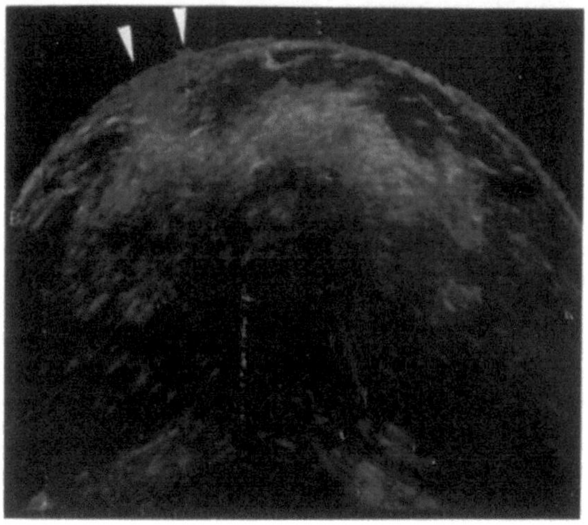

d

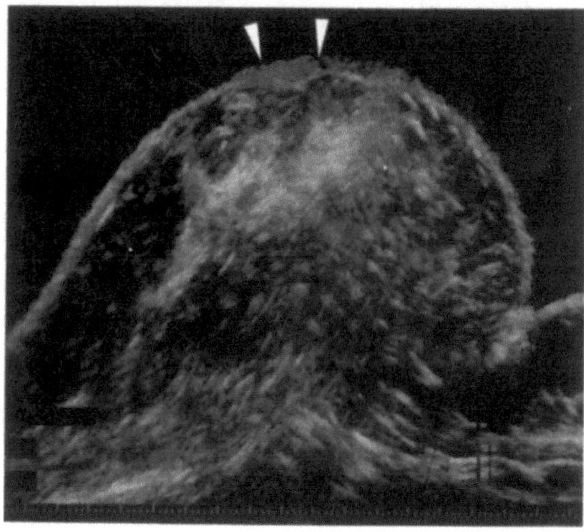

e

Fig. 5.4a-e. Inflammatory carcinoma. Sonogram shows thickened, mottled, doubly contoured skin layer. The lower contour is disrupted at several points

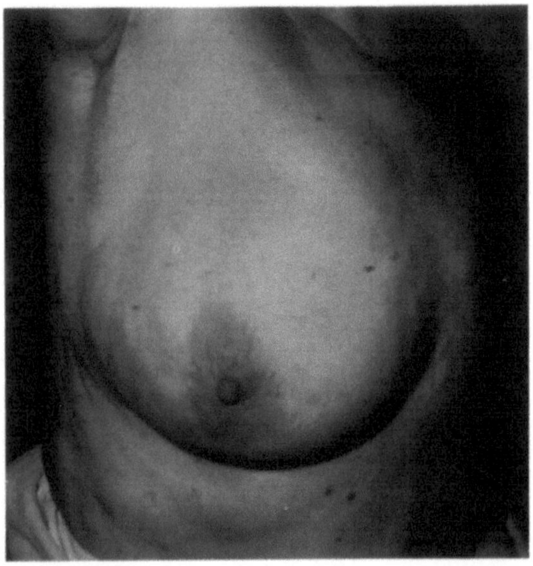
a

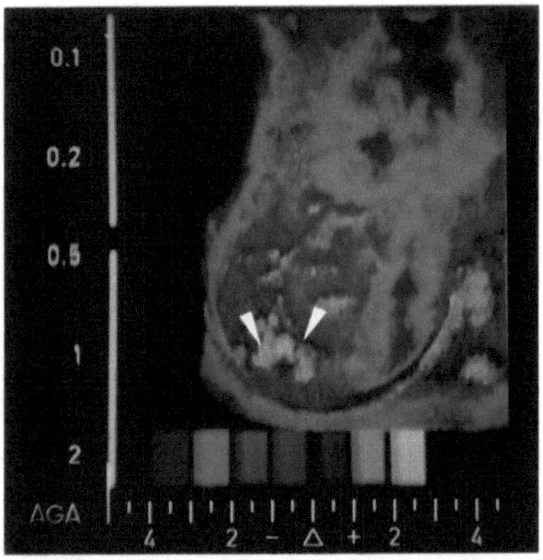

b

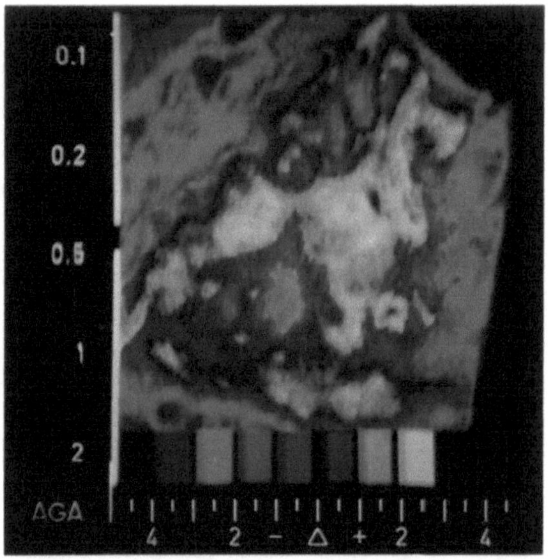

c

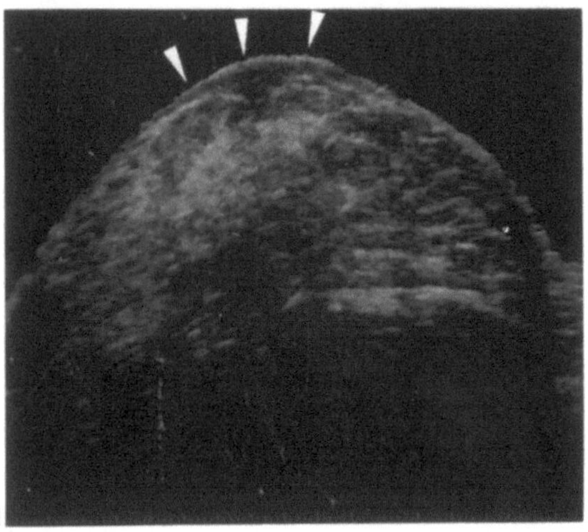
d

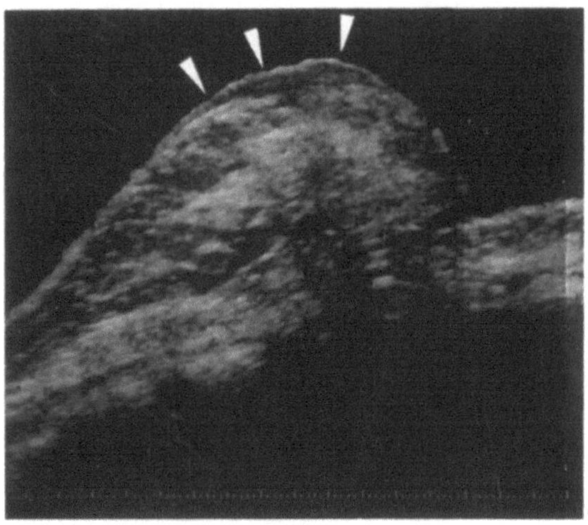
e

Sonography Versus X-Ray Mammography

Next to physical examination, X-ray mammography is the oldest diagnostic method for evaluations of the breast. In preparation for X-ray mammography, compression is applied to the breast to immobilize it, to equalize the thicknesses of the basal and peripheral breast areas, and to reduce scatter radiation, which increases with the thickness of the organ being examined. The summation-type images are ordinarily taken in the craniocaudal and mediolateral projections. Axillary and magnification films also may be obtained. The mammogram should cover the entire breast including the retromammary space and axillary extension. The X-ray beam should always strike the nipple tangentially, and the axilla and associated lymph nodes should be depicted at least on the axillary film.

The glandular parenchyma, fat, connective tissue, milk ducts, and blood vessels of the breast differ very little in their capacities for X-ray absorption. Hence special techniques must be used to ensure an optimum reproduction of breast anatomy and morphology (Table 5.2).

Recent advances in mammographic imaging have made it possible to reduce the mid-breast dose for a standard two-view examination to 0.35 to 0.40 rad, implying an extremely low risk of mammographically induced carcinogenesis. This technical advance is certainly due in part to public anxiety about the harmful effects of X-rays, but it also relates to the advent of new diagnostic modalities, such as sonography, that do not involve exposure to ionizing radiation.

As in sonography, the evaluation of X-ray mammograms relies on the use of various interpretive criteria (Table 5.3).

Recommendations on the use of X-ray mammography have come from numerous sources. One of the most authoritative is Bastert and colleagues (1985), who were commissioned by the German Cancer Society and the Association of German Tumor Centers (Table 5.4).

Besides areas in which sonography and X-ray mammography yield comparable results, there are special areas in which one of the modalities is superior to the other (Table 5.5).

Table 5.2. Modern X-Ray mammographic techniques.

Low-kilovoltage ("soft beam") technique (e.g., molybdenum target with 25–30 kV energies, 32 kV maximum)
X-ray beam filtering with a beryllium-molybdenum sheet to maintain a lower beam energy
Special moving grid for enhanced image contrast and detail
Fixed focus-film distance (60 cm, "long cone" technique)
Automatic timer to ensure constant film exposure
High-definition film-screen combinations (reduce necessary exposure by 50% or more compared with dose previously required)

Table 5.3. Interpretive criteria in X-ray mammography.

1. Circumscribed architectural changes
   - Connective tissue proliferation
   - Periductal fibrosis
2. Circumscribed densities (opacities)
   - Uniformly or nonuniformly radiopaque
   - Faint
   - Smooth or partially smooth margins (0.7% and 15%, respectively, of all carcinomas; Barth, 1977)
   - Ill-defined margins and radial projections
   - "Stellate" density
3. Calcifications
   - Moderately radiolucent, rounded, nonclustered
     - In glandular tissue (small calcified cysts)
     - In subcutaneous fat layer (oil cysts associated with fat necrosis)
     - In skin (sebaceous cysts)
   - Often bizarre, coarse, occurring within densities (calcified fibroadenoma)
   - Lancet-shaped, following the course of milk ducts (plasma cell mastitis)
   - Rodlike (small calcified arteries)
   - Clustered (at least 10–15 foci), polymorphous, densely radiopaque, 1–100 μm in size (suspicious for malignancy)
4. Other abnormalities
   - Skin changes (thickening, reticular or striate mottling, retraction)
   - Nipple changes (retraction, retroareolar abnormalities)
   - Abnormal venous pattern (large-caliber veins arising from densities)

Table 5.4. Recommendations for the use of X-ray mammography.

Women not at high risk for breast carcinoma	
	Baseline mammogram at age 35–40
	Two-year follow-ups from age 40 to 65
Women at high risk for breast carcinoma	
	Baseline mammogram at age 25–30
	1 to 1½-year follow-ups from age 30 to 65

From Bastert et al., 1985.

Table 5.5. Values of ultrasound and X-ray mammography in different diagnostic settings.

Diagnostic situation	Ultrasound	X-ray mammography
Pregnancy	+	−
Peripheral lesions	+	(+) to −
Bedridden patients	+	− to (+)
Cystic/solid differentiation	+	−
Abscess detection in mastitis	+	−
Evaluation of prostheses	+	(+)
Dense breast	+	(+) to −
Involuted breast	(+) to −	+
Microcalcifications	− to (+)	+
Intraductal masses	−	+ (ductography)
Examination of surgical specimens	(+)	+

Table 5.6. Accuracy rates of ultrasound (US) and X-ray mammography in carcinoma diagnosis.

Carcinomas of all sizes (260 = 100%)	US +[a]	US −
	245 (94%)	15 (6%)
X-ray + 248 (95%)	235 (90%)	13 (5%)
X-ray − 12 (5%)	10 (4%)	2 (1%)
Carcinomas ≤ cm (39 = 100%)	32 (82%)	7 (18%)
X-ray + 36 (92%)	30 (77%)	6 (15%)
X-ray − 3 (8%)	2 (5%)	1 (3%)

[a] +, positive; −, negative.

Peripheral lesions that are poorly accessible to X-ray mammography cause no difficulty whatsoever in breast sonography. The same is true for bed-confined patients (Fig. 5.5). Ultrasound offers an alternative in situations such as pregnancy (Fig. 5.6), where exposure to ionizing radiation is not desired, and in "radiophobic" patients who will not submit to X-ray examination. The differentiation of cystic and solid masses and the detection of abscesses (as in mastitis) have been considered the domain of ultrasound all along (Fig. 5.7, 5.8).

"Pneumocystography" is an important adjunct to sonographic cyst diagnosis and the ultrasound-guided aspiration of cystic masses. While air insufflation into an aspirated cyst prevents further evaluation of the area with ultrasound, it serves as a prophylaxis against cyst refilling, and high-quality radiographic images can be taken showing the margination and degree of emptying of the cyst. Occasionally, the increased transparency produced by air injection allows portions of the breast to be visualized more clearly than on plain radiographs.

The evaluation of breast implants and residual tissue, difficult with radiography, can be easily accomplished with ultrasound (Chap. 4, Figs. 4.8–4.11, 5.9).

While sonography is superior to radiography in the evaluation of dense breasts (Fig. 5.10), radiographs yield more information in the involuted breast (Fig. 5.11). Both modalities yield comparably good results in the diagnosis of breast carcinoma, although tumors up to 1 cm in diameter are detected more reliably with X-rays (92%) than with ultrasound (82%). With the combined application of both modalities, only 1% of all carcinomas are missed, and only 3% of carcinomas up to 1 cm in size (Table 5.6).

Microcalcifications

Clustered microcalcifications are considered the most important suggestive sign of neoplasia in X-ray mammography. Different authors ascribe different levels of significance to the phenomenon. While Lanyi (1985) found microcalcifications as the sole evidence of malignancy in 50 of 519 breast carcinomas followed for approximately 10 years, a screening study by Lundgren (1979) in Sweden found that only 2.3% of all carcinomas were detected on the basis of microcalcifications alone.

In the past, microcalcifications were thought to be undetectable with ultrasound. It was assumed that while microcalcifications indeed produce echoes on sonograms, it would not be possible to identify these echoes as calcific foci (Fig. 5.12). This view is being challenged, however, by the latest generation of ultrasound instruments, which make use of computer-controlled transducer technology. Initial experience with these systems suggests that they are capable of demonstrating microcalcifications reproducibly (Figs. 5.13, 5.14).

Radiography is unquestionably superior to sonography in the evaluation of the mammary ducts by contrast ductography (see Chap. 2; Figs. 2.1, 5.15). The reported detection rate of carcinomas by ductography alone is on the order of 2 to 4% (Frischbier and Lohbeck, 1977; Kindermann, 1985). Less importance is attached to the gross examination of nipple discharge and to the cytologic evaluation of breast smears. In selected cases sonography and ductography can be excellent complements to each other in evaluation of the mammary ducts.

In principle, both sonography and radiography can be used to examine surgical specimens (Fig. 5.16). Radiography is the method of choice, however, owing to its practicability and the relative ease of examining tissue pieces containing microcalcifications.

Screening

While screening studies in the United States, Holland, Sweden, and West Germany in recent years have established the value of X-ray mammography, breast ultrasound has so far been tested as a screening procedure only in Japan, but with positive results (Table 5.7).

Sonographic Guidance of Needle Aspirations and Biopsies

The sonographic criteria described for cysts in Chapter 2 – smooth margins, echo-free interior, posterior enhancement, intracystic structures – can be confirmed with ultrasound before an aspiration is performed. With pre-aspiration radiography, cysts appear only as faint, more or less well-circumscribed densities, and a more accurate assessment requires that a pneumocystogram be taken after the aspiration is completed (Fig. 5.17). The advantage of sonographic guidance for cyst aspiration is that it enables direct monitoring of the aspiration procedure. The aspirating needle can be directed with precision; often an unsuccessful aspiration can be seen to be caused by the needle's impressing on the cyst wall without penetrating it (Fig. 5.18a,b). An incomplete evacuation is easily recognized and can be corrected without delay (Fig. 5.18c). A complete evacuation is indicated by disappearance of the mass from the scan (Fig. 5.18d). Subsequent air injection to inhibit cyst refill and prepare for pneumocystography creates a total acoustic barrier that renders the area invisible to ultrasound (Fig. 5.19d). The presumptive volume of material to be aspirated from the cyst can be estimated beforehand by determining the mean cyst radius or diameter on three planes and then applying the formula for the volume of a sphere ($4/3 \cdot \pi \cdot r^3$) (Table 5.8).

Ultrasound is also able to demonstrate the location of the needle used to biopsy a solid breast mass (Fig. 5.20). As in the aspiration of cystic masses, it is possible with ultrasound to correct the needle placement while the biopsy is being performed. With radiographic guidance (Fig. 5.21), on the other hand, it is necessary to interrupt the biopsy procedure, and the compression that is applied may cause displacement of the needle. Of course, the value of radiographic localization remains undisputed for lesions that are sonographically occult (Fig. 5.22).

Given these facts and the capabilities of sonographic needle guidance, we feel that the technique of stereotaxic breast biopsy under radiographic vision using the Nordenström apparatus is too costly and time consuming to be justified (Bolmgren et al., 1977; Nordenström and Zajicek, 1977). More recent stereotaxic apparatus, such as the Thomson CGR unit released in 1988, is currently undergoing clinical evaluation.

The indications for sonography and radiography in breast aspirations and biopsies, and the places of these modalities in the diagnosis of breast disease, are summarized in Tables 5.9 and 5.10.

Table 5.7. Breast screening projects.

Study	Period	Screening methods, technical aspects	Population	Results
Miyagi Prefecture, Japan (Abe et al., 1985)	Since 1977	X-ray mammography plus ultrasound (US)	90,076 women	Carcinoma detection rate, 0.12%; detection rate of small tumors increases, rate of lymph node metastasis declines
Toyama Prefecture, Japan (Wagai and Tsutsumi, 1983)	Since 1975 Since 1981	Clinical exam plus US (mechanical linear scanner) Clinical exam plus US (immersion scanner)	29,673 women by 1982	Carcinoma detection rate, 0.06%
Kouchi Screening Clinic, Japan (Kobayashi, 1983)	1979–1982	Clinical exam plus US	6031 women	Carcinoma detection rate, 0.06%
HIP study (Health Insurance Plan, New York); USA (Feig, 1985)	1963–1970	Clinical exam plus biplane X-rays, yearly (randomized study)	2 groups of 31,000 women age 40–64	Detection rate: Carcinomas $\leq$ 1 cm and in situ carcinomas, 8% Mortality reduction: ~20–30% (significant only for women over age 50)
BCDDP (Breast Cancer Detection Demonstration Project), USA (Feig, 1985)	1973–1981	Clinical exam plus biplane X-rays	~300,000 women	Detection rate: Carcinomas $\leq$ 1 cm and in situ carcinomas, 36% Mortality reduction: > 50% for women of all ages
Utrecht Project (DOM), Holland (Feig, 1985)	Since 1974	Clinical exam plus biplane X-rays, follow-up at 12, 18, and 24 months	~15,000 women age 50–64	Mortality reduction: ca. 70%
Nijmegen Project, Holland (Feig, 1985)	1975–1982	X-rays on one plane only; four follow-ups at 2-yr intervals	30,000 women age 35–65	Mortality reduction: ca. 50% (significant for women over age 55)
Kopparberg-Östergötland Project, Sweden (Feig, 1985)	1977–1984	Only one "medio-lateral" X-ray, radomized study	162,981 women age 40 or older	Mortality reduction: > 40% Reduction of tumors > T_2
Hamburg Screening Program, FRG (Frischbier, 1985)	Since 1971	Biplane X-rays every 2 years, controlled prospective study	14,002 clinically normal women by end of 1984	Increase of in situ carcinomas and tumors without demonstrable lymph node metastases Reduction of T_1 and T_2 tumors 5-yr survival rate: 96% in screened group (n=102), 57% in controls (n=276) (between 1970 and 1976)

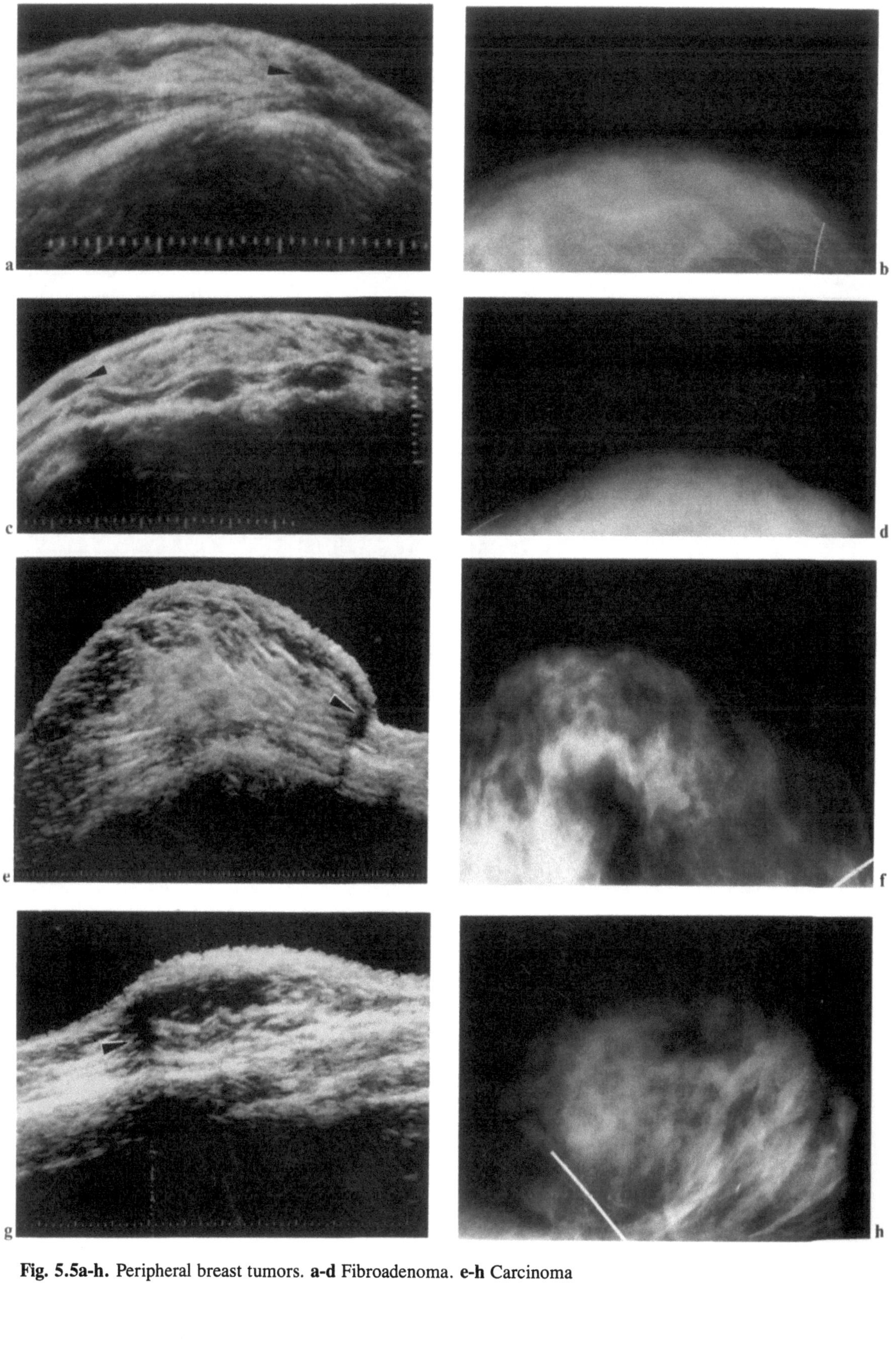

Fig. 5.5a-h. Peripheral breast tumors. **a-d** Fibroadenoma. **e-h** Carcinoma

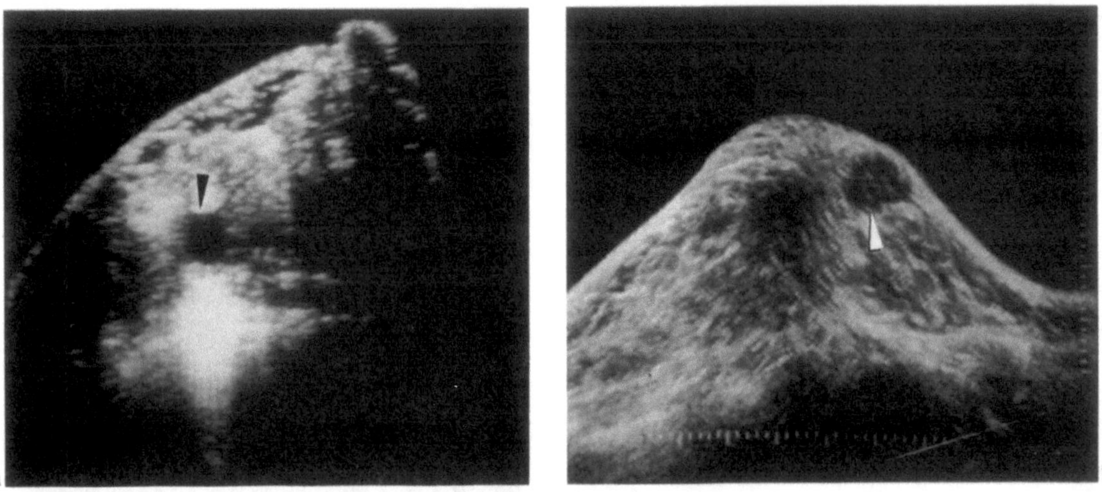

a b

Fig. 5.6a,b. Focal masses in pregnancy. **a** Cyst in a 42-year-old woman in the 15th week of pregnancy. **b** Fibroadenoma in a 26-year-old woman in the 16th week of pregnancy

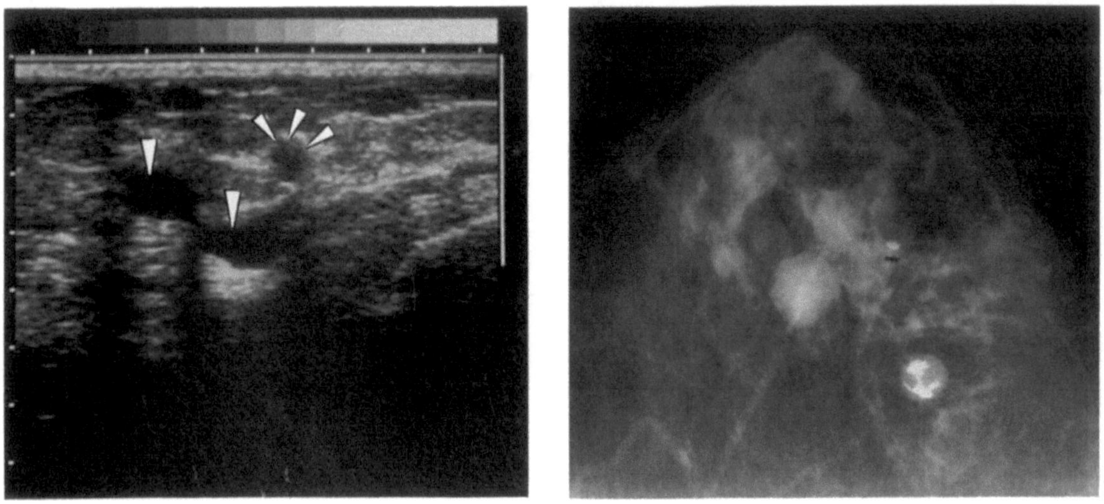

a b

Fig. 5.7a,b. Sonogram (**a**) demonstrates two cystic masses and one solid mass, and radiograph (**b**) discloses multiple densities, some showing coarse calcification

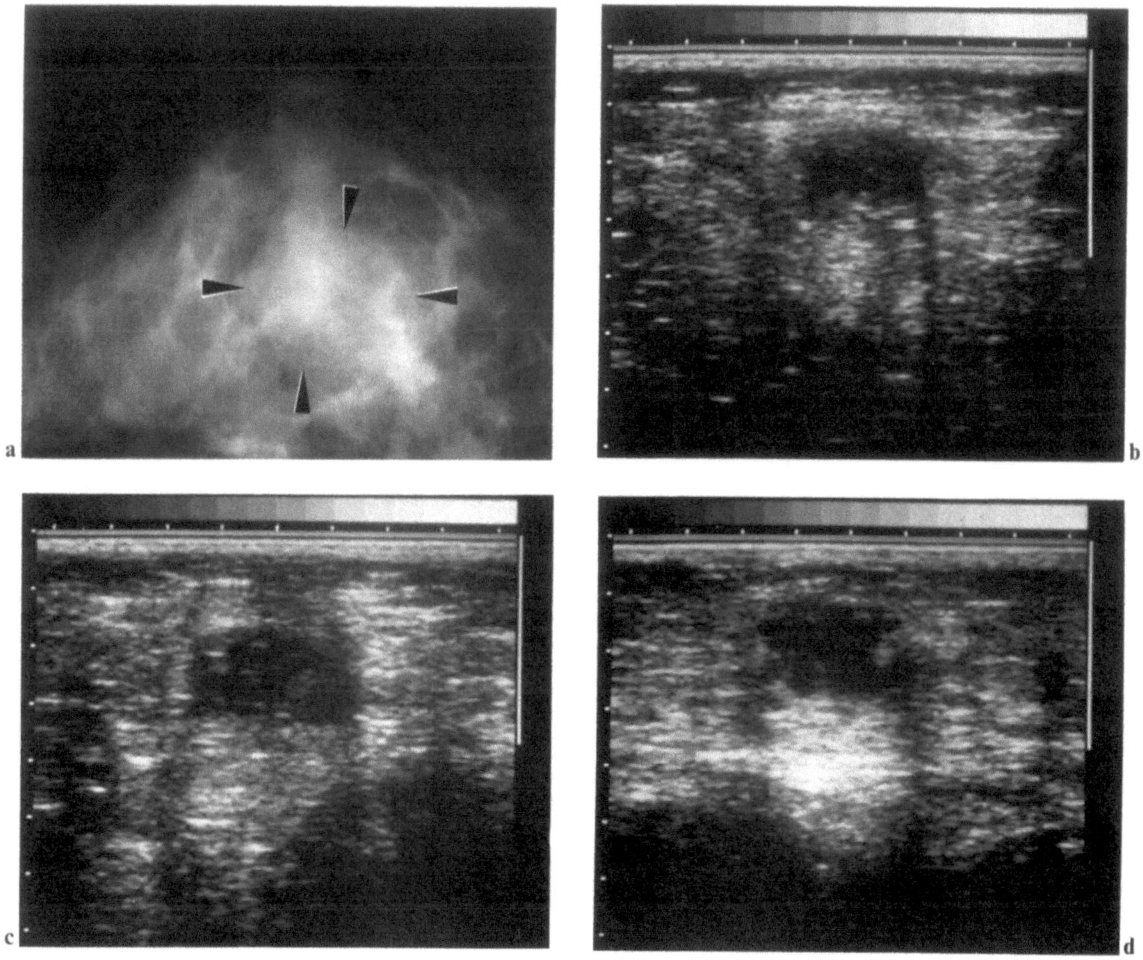

Fig. 5.8a-d. Radiographic density in the breast parenchyma of a 34-year-old woman (**a**). Initial sonogram shows ill-defined hypoechoic lesion (**b**) that appears markedly enlarged 2 days later (**c**) and t days later casts a dense posterior enhancement (**d**). Incision of the breast at that time disclosed nonpuerperal mastitis with abscess formation

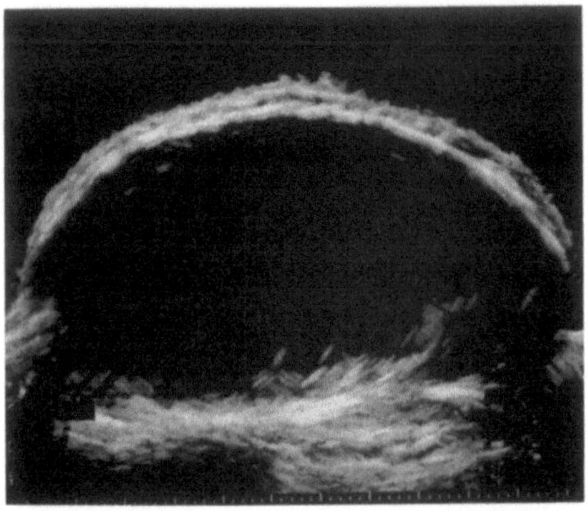
a

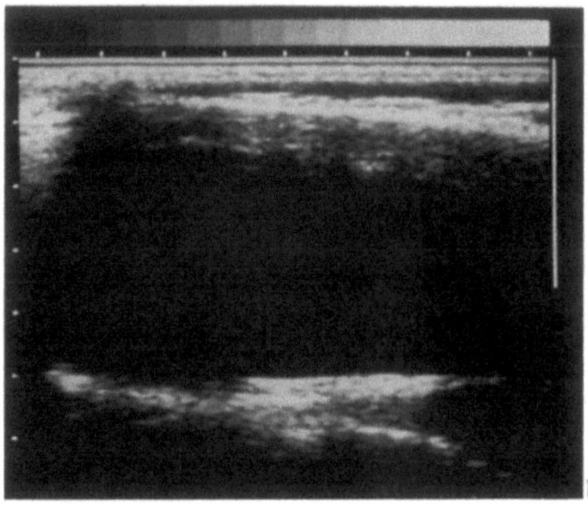
b

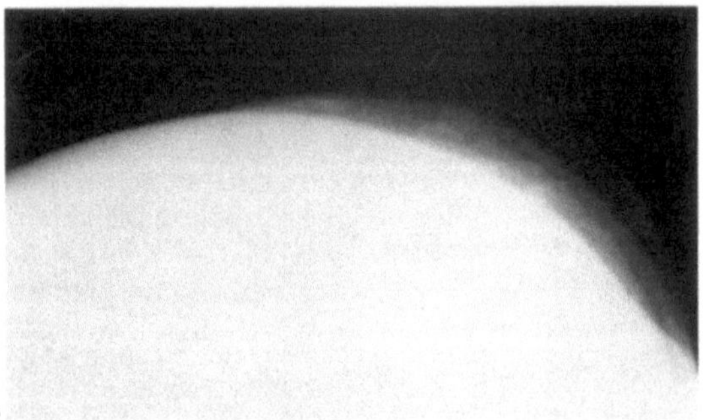
c

Fig. 5.9a-c. Breast prosthesis. **a** The anterior wall is very well delineated on the immersion scan. **b** The posterior wall is shown better on the contact scan. **c** The radiograph gives virtually no useful information

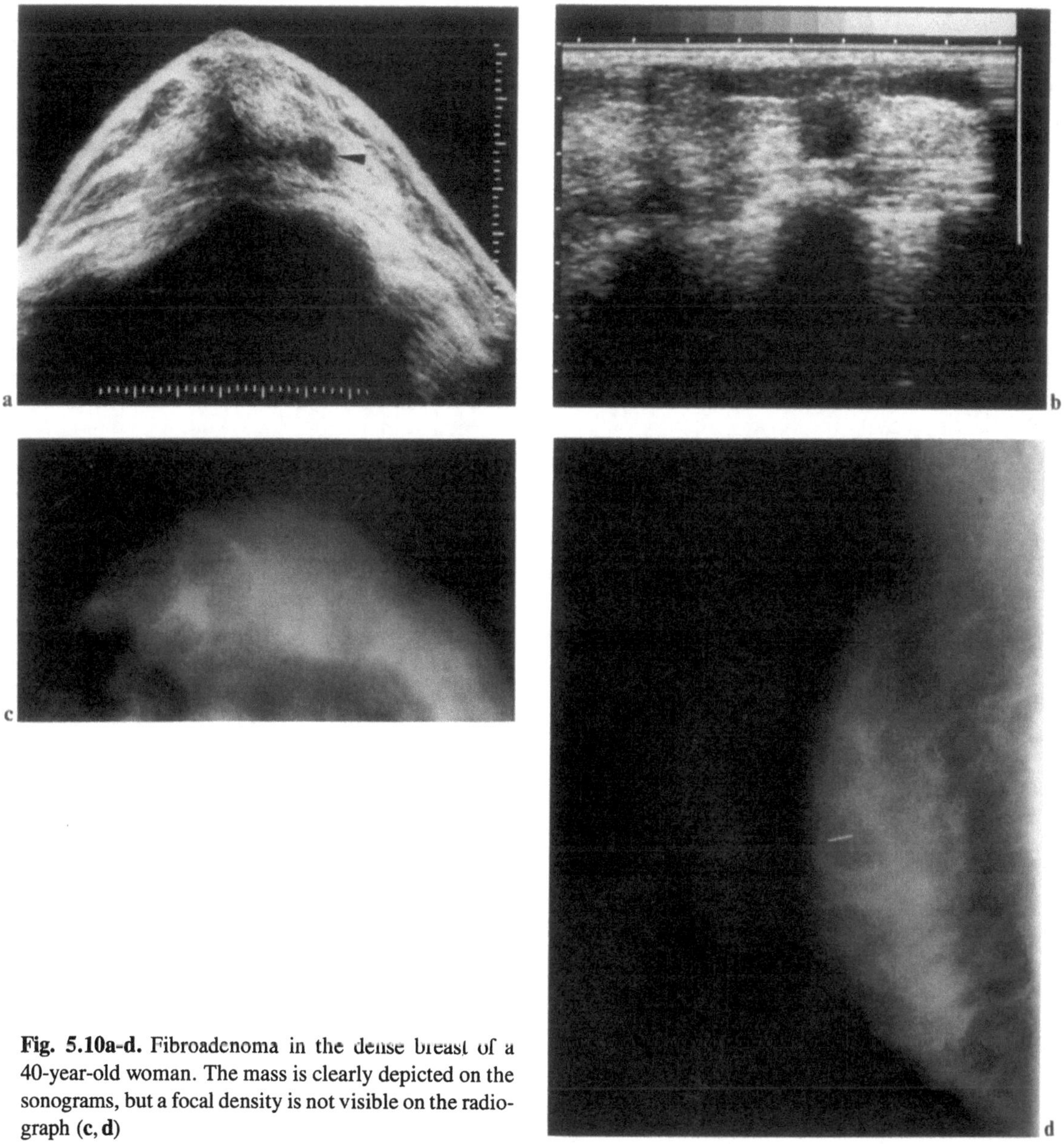

Fig. 5.10a-d. Fibroadenoma in the dense breast of a 40-year-old woman. The mass is clearly depicted on the sonograms, but a focal density is not visible on the radiograph (**c, d**)

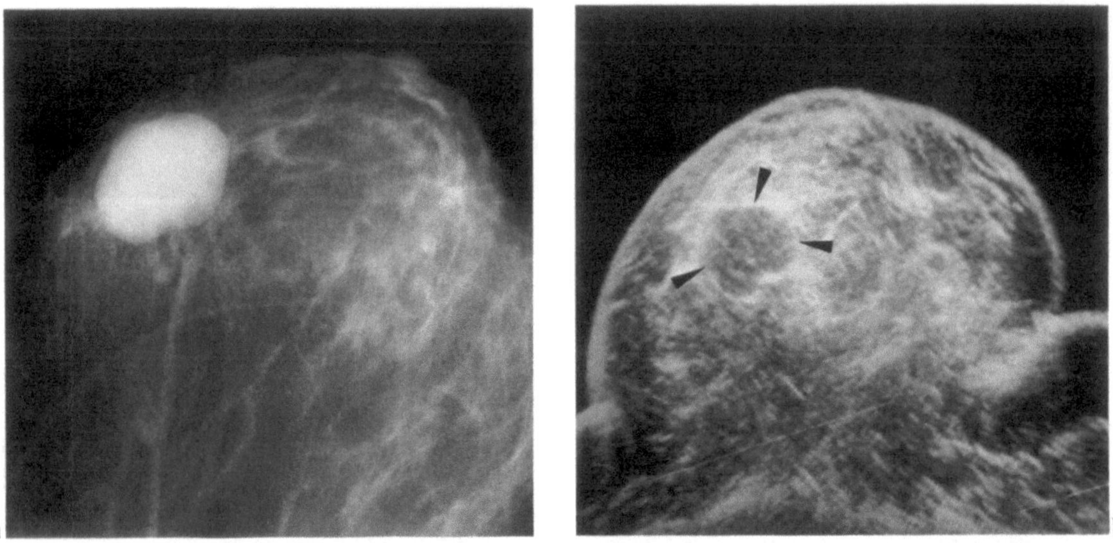

Fig. 5.11a,b. Fibroadenoma in the involuted breast of a 43-year-old woman. The well-circumscribed density is conspicuous on the radiograph (**a**), but the sonographic lesion (**b**) is barely distinguishable from involuted tissue

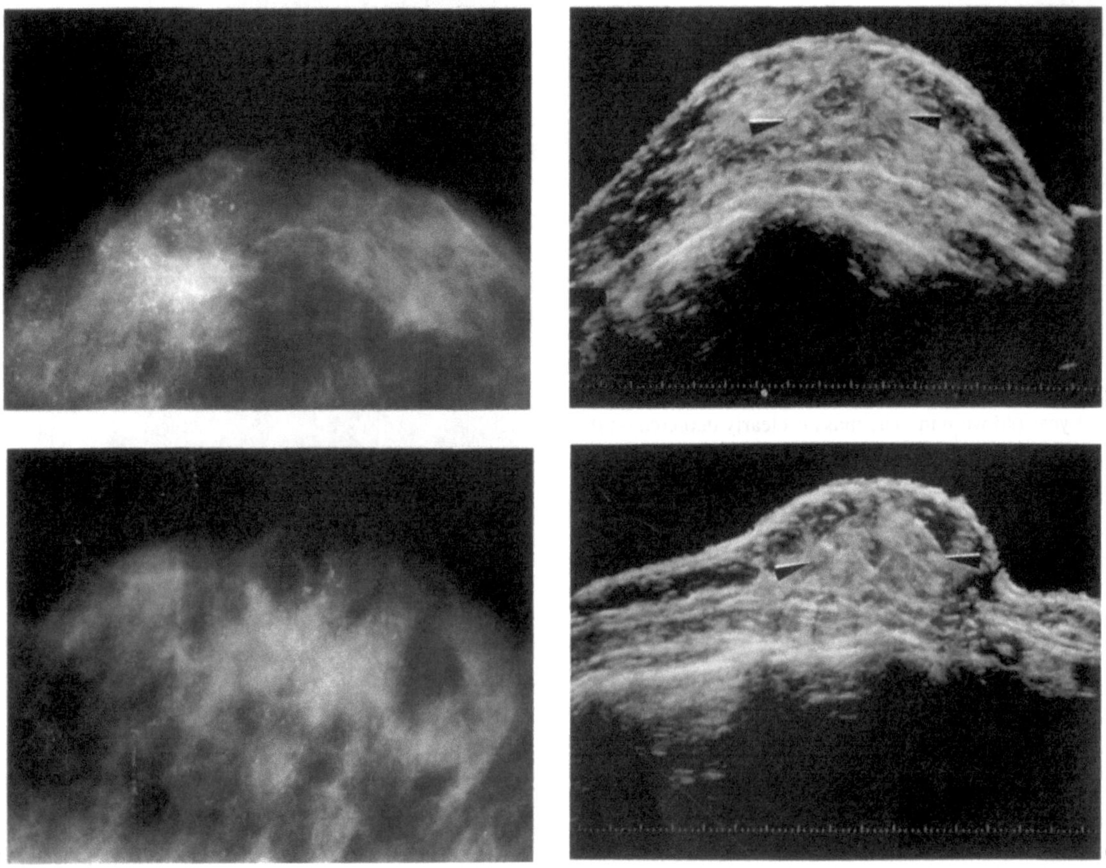

Fig. 5.12a-d. Diffuse microcalcifications in a 47-year-old woman with a 3×2.5-cm predominantly intraductal comedocarcinoma. The microcalcifications seen on the X-rays (**a,c**) are not represented on the sonograms (**b,d**)

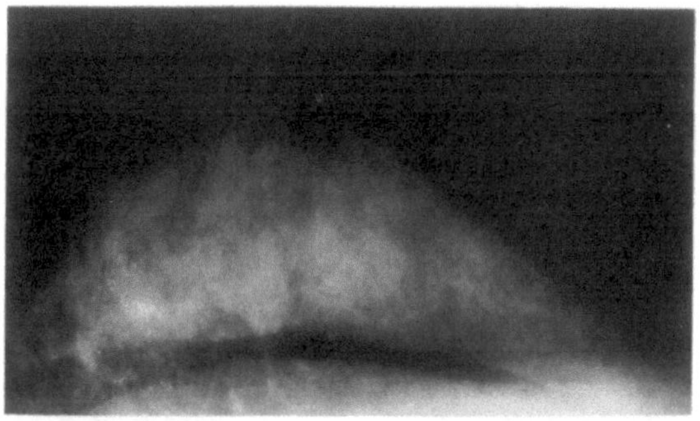
a

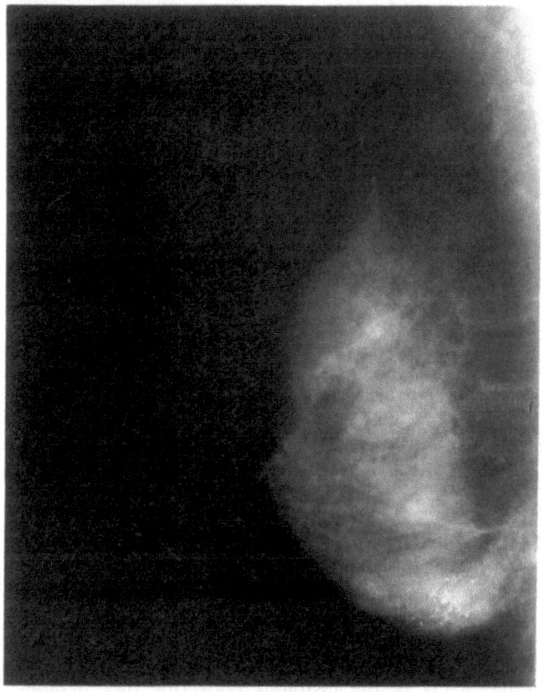
b

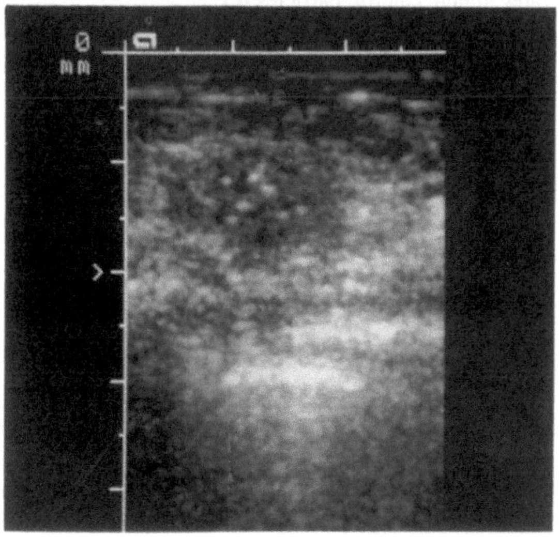
c

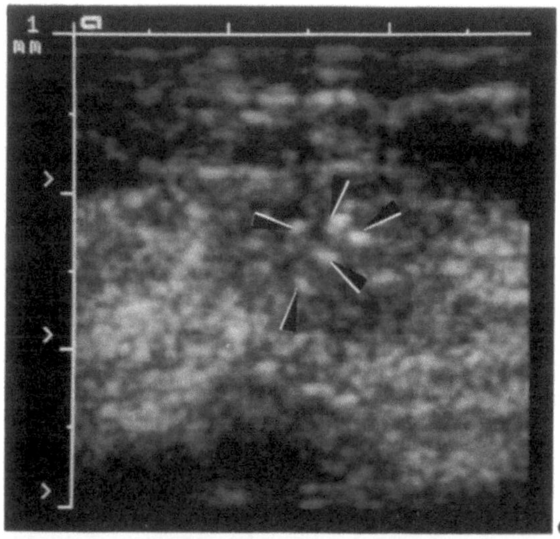
d

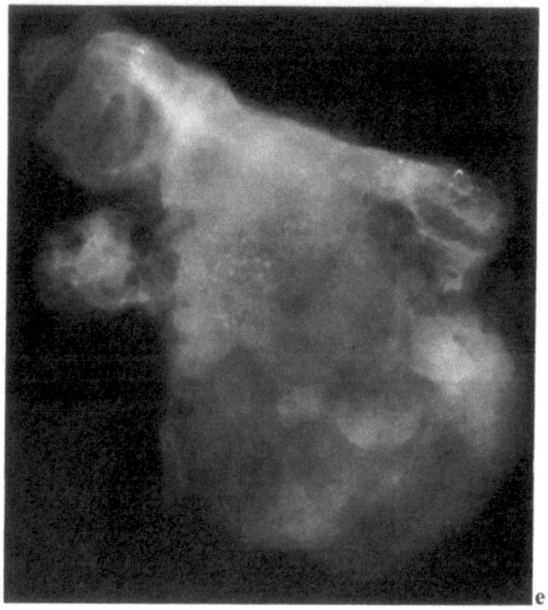
e

Fig. 5.13a-e. Clustered microcalcifications in a 54-year-old woman with extensive intraductal comedocarcinoma. Sonogram (**c,d**) shows a 1.7×1.3-cm mass with multiple high-level punctate echoes that apparently represent microcalcifications. Radiograph (**a,b,e**) confirms (**e**) that the focus of calcification is included in the specimen (**e**)

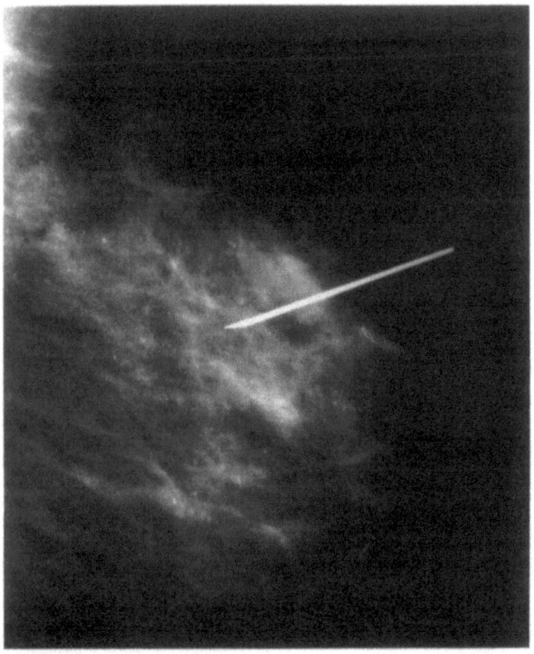

a

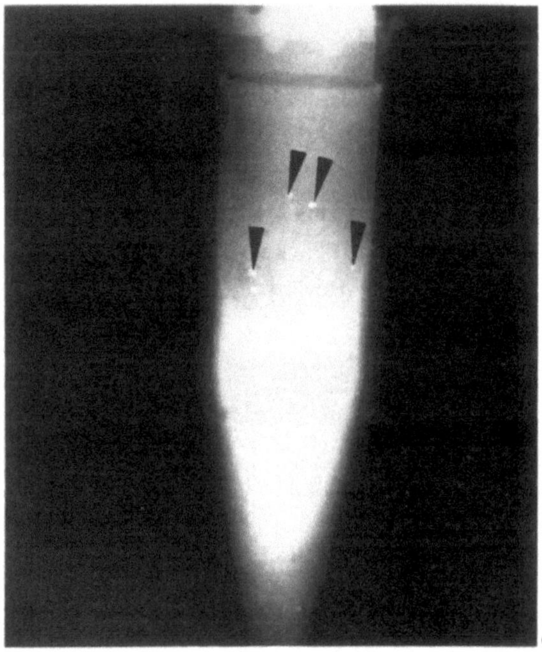

c

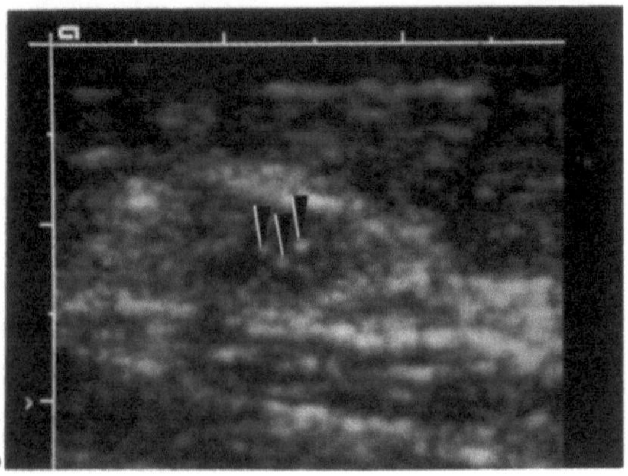

b

Fig. 5.14a-c. Diffuse clustered microcalcifications in a 48-year-old woman with a 2.5×2-cm intraductal carcinoma and a 1-cm carcinoma with invasive components. The mass is nonpalpable, and X-rays show only the calcifications. Ultrasound **(a,b)** shows a 1-cm hypoechoic mass with high-level punctate echoes. Needle biopsy of the sonographic lesion discloses a Papanicolaou class V cytology and the histologic picture of invasive carcinoma. X-ray of the histology collecting tube demonstrates minute calcific particles **(c)**

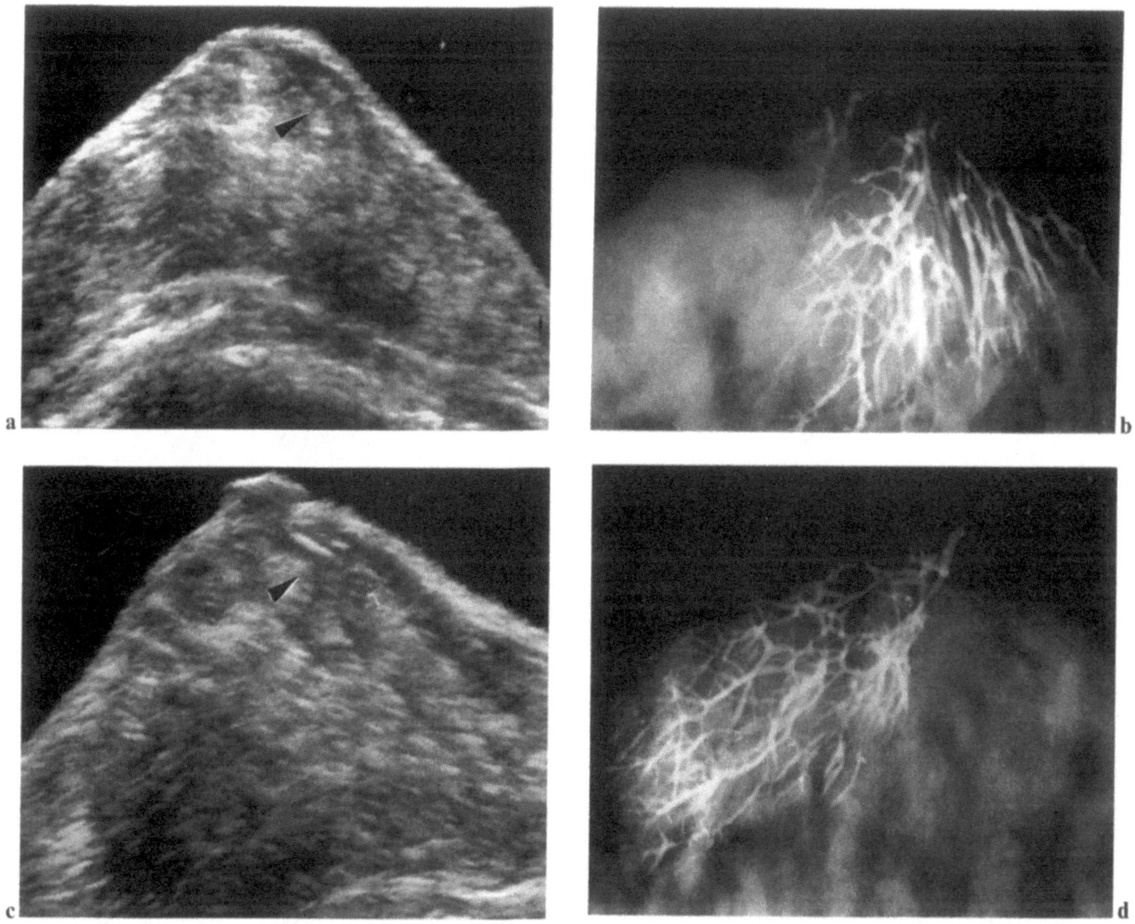

Fig. 5.15a-d. 31-year-old woman with bloody nipple discharge in the 34th week of pregnancy. Sonograms (**a,c**) show ductectasia in the right lower inner breast quadrant. Subsequent contrast ductography (**b,d**) localizes the secreting duct to the upper inner quadrant

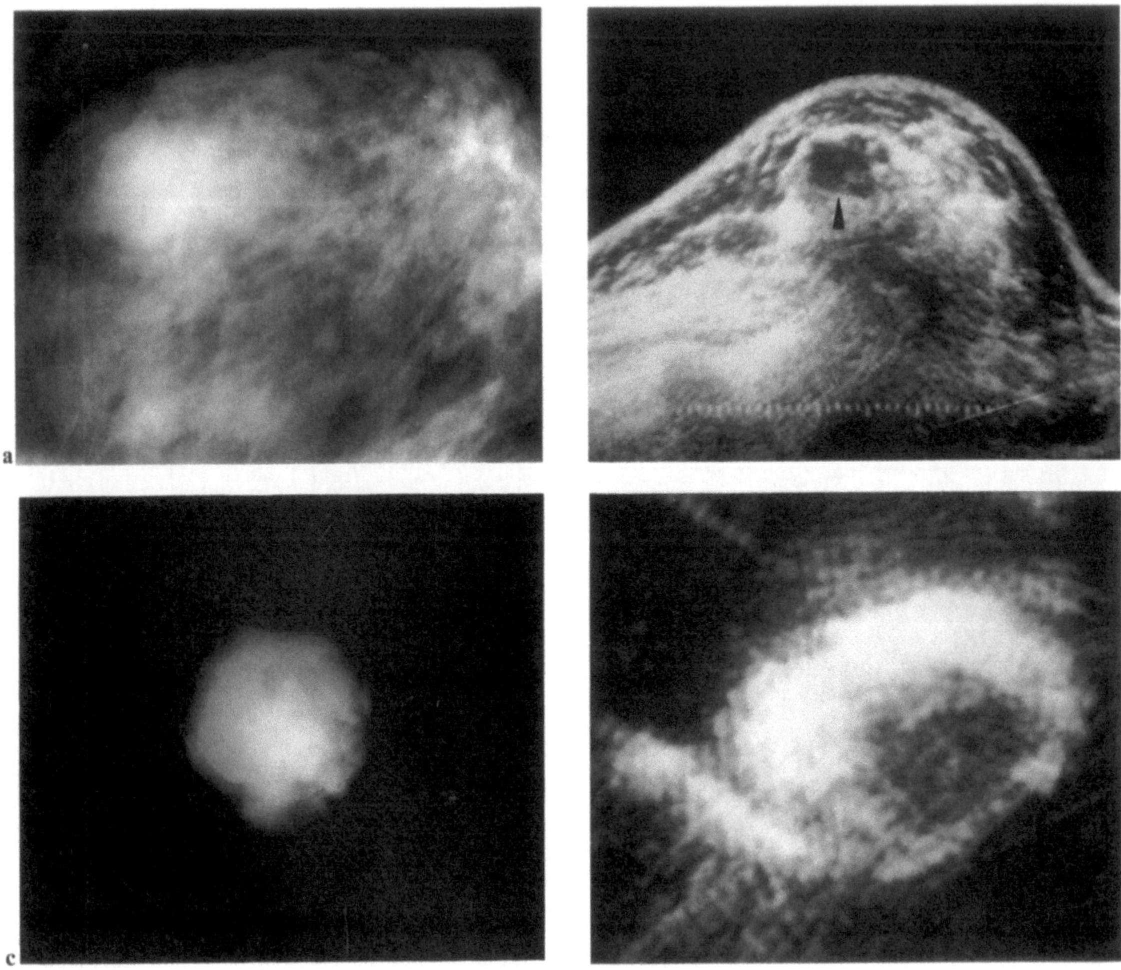

Fig. 5.16a-d. Radiographically and sonographically demonstrable mass (**a,b**) in a 47-year-old woman. Specimen radiograph (**c**) and specimen sonogram (**d**) after tumor excision. Histology identified the lesion as a circumscribed area of grade II fibrocystic disease

Table 5.8. Cyst diameter versus internal volume.

Mean cyst diameter (cm)	Presumptive volume of cyst content (ml)
1	0.5
2	4.2
3	14.2
4	33.5
5	65.5

Table 5.9. Indications for sonographically or radiographically guided fine-needle aspirations of the breast.

Sonography	Radiography
General	General
All sonographic focal lesions, especially when accompanied by palpable mass, mammographic abnormality, or other correlate	All lesions inaccessible or poorly accessible to ultrasound imaging (e.g., clustered microcalcifications)
Special	Special
Nonpalpable lesions	Cysts that have been aspirated and filled with air (PCG[a])
Lesions inaccessible or poorly accessible to radiographic imaging, especially in dense breast	
Breast lesions in pregnancy	
Peripherally located masses not demonstrated clearly or completely by radiography	
Masses in bed-confined patients	

[a] PCG, pneumocytography.

Table 5.10. Role of sonographically guided breast aspirations and biopsies compared with those guided by radiography.

Feature	Ultrasound	Radiography
Ability to visualize mass prior to aspiration or biopsy	Cystic/solid differentiation, margins, internal echoes, secondary phenomena	Margins, microcalcifications
Ability to visualize mass during aspiration or biopsy	Good	Not possible
Control of needle placement	Dynamic, direct, painless, does not affect needle placement	Static, delays needle placement, can be painful, often alters needle placement
Correction of needle placement	Permits immediate correction	Does not permit immediate correction
Ability to visualize mass following aspiration or biopsy	Cysts: good before air filling, not possible afterward	Cysts: pneumocystography (very good)
	Solid masses: good	Solid masses: good
Guidance of needle into nonpalpable mass	Can be done without difficulty	Uncertain
Radiation exposure	None	Present
Documentation costs	For 1 (or 2) sonograms	For 2 (up to 4) radiographs (plain film plus PCG or needle placement, 2 views each)

PCG, pneumocystography.

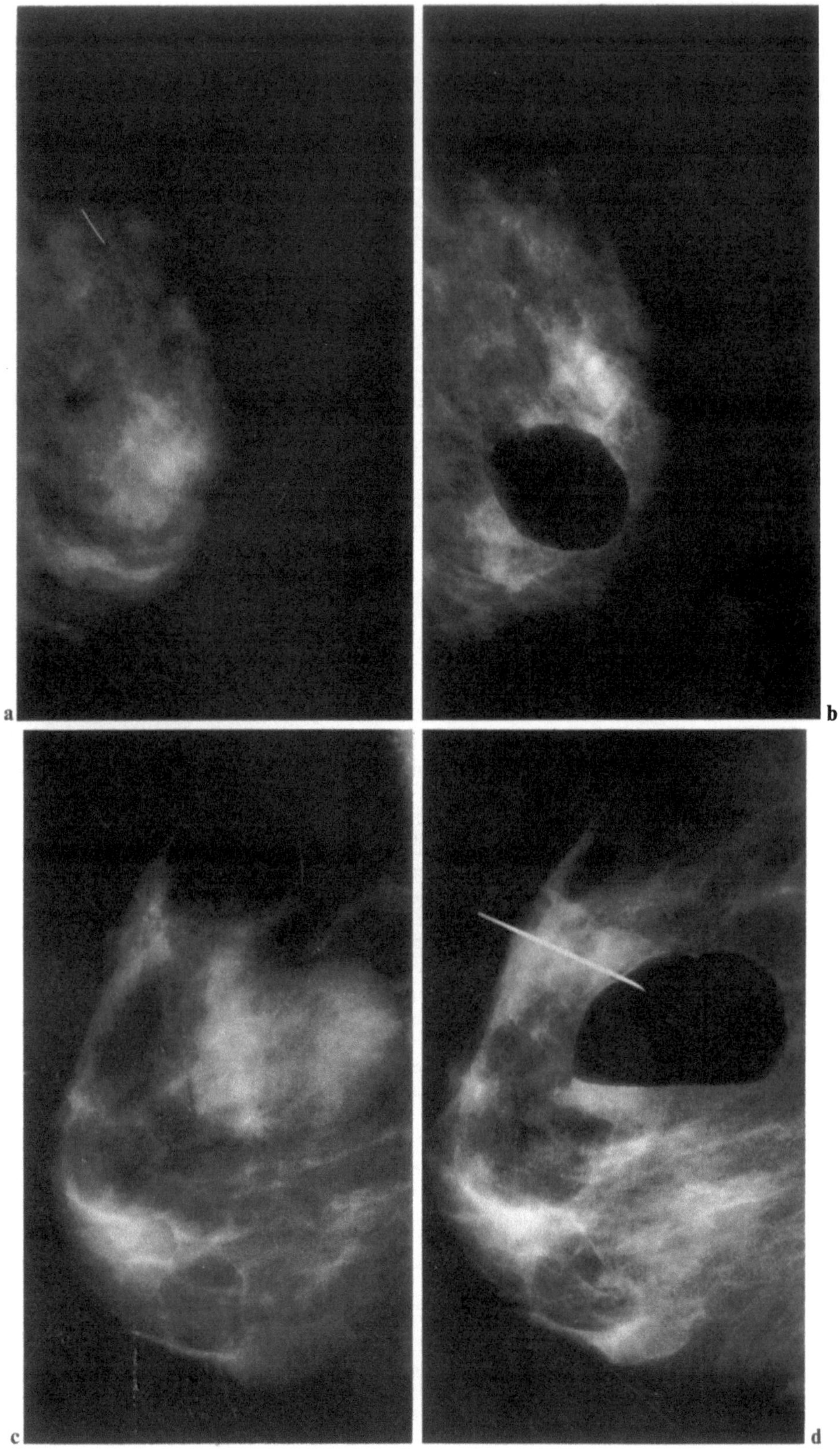

Fig. 5.17a-f. Pneumocystograms. **a,b** Completely evaluated cyst with smooth margins. **c,d** Incompletely evacuated cyst with fluid level. **e,f** Intracystic carcinoma

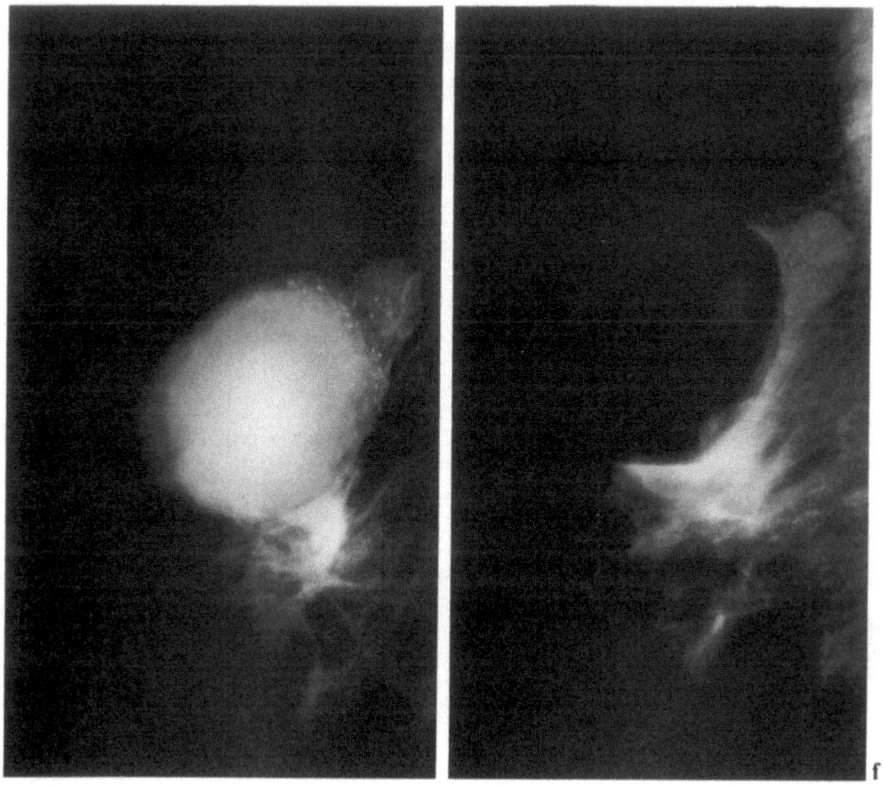

e f

Fig. 5.17e-f.

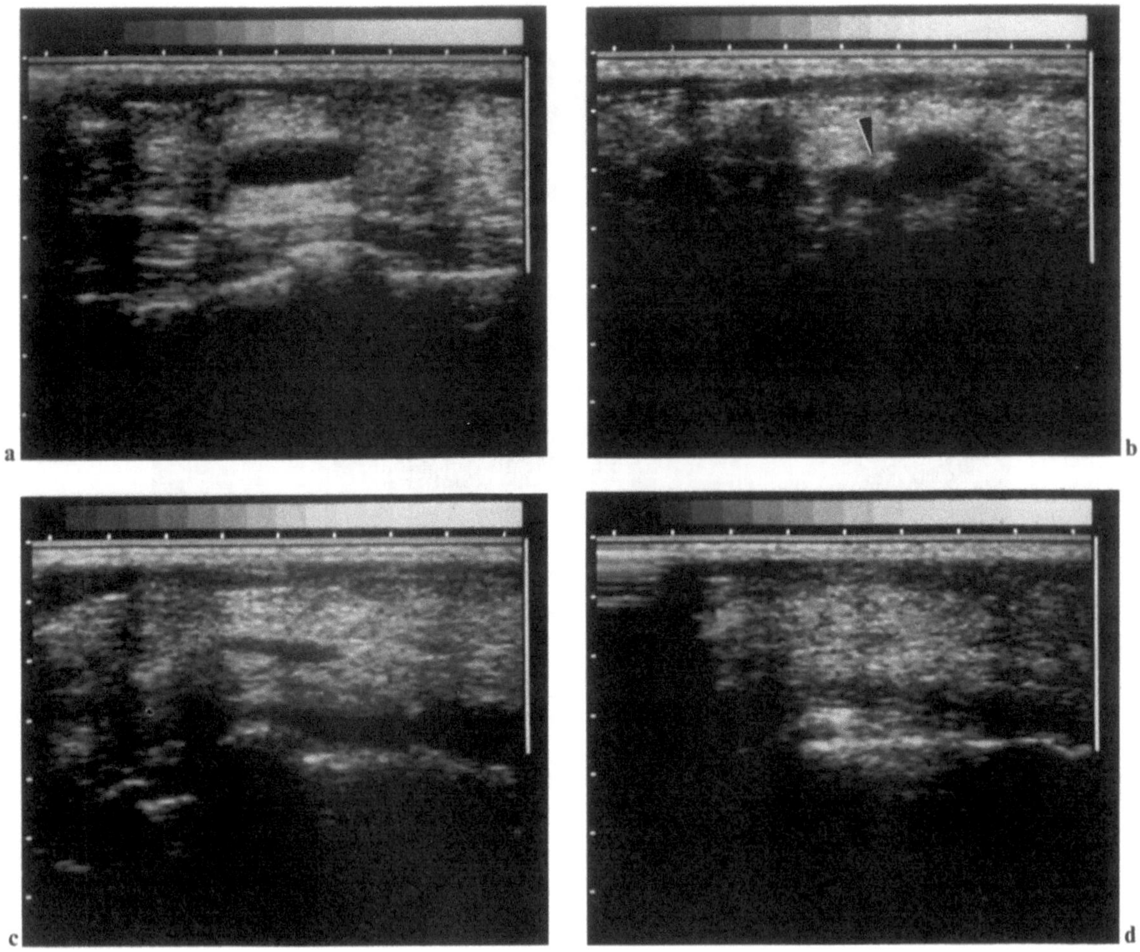

Fig. 5.18. **a** Cyst prior to aspiration. **b** Aspirating needle indenting the cyst wall. **c** Partially evacuated cyst. **d** Evacuated cyst

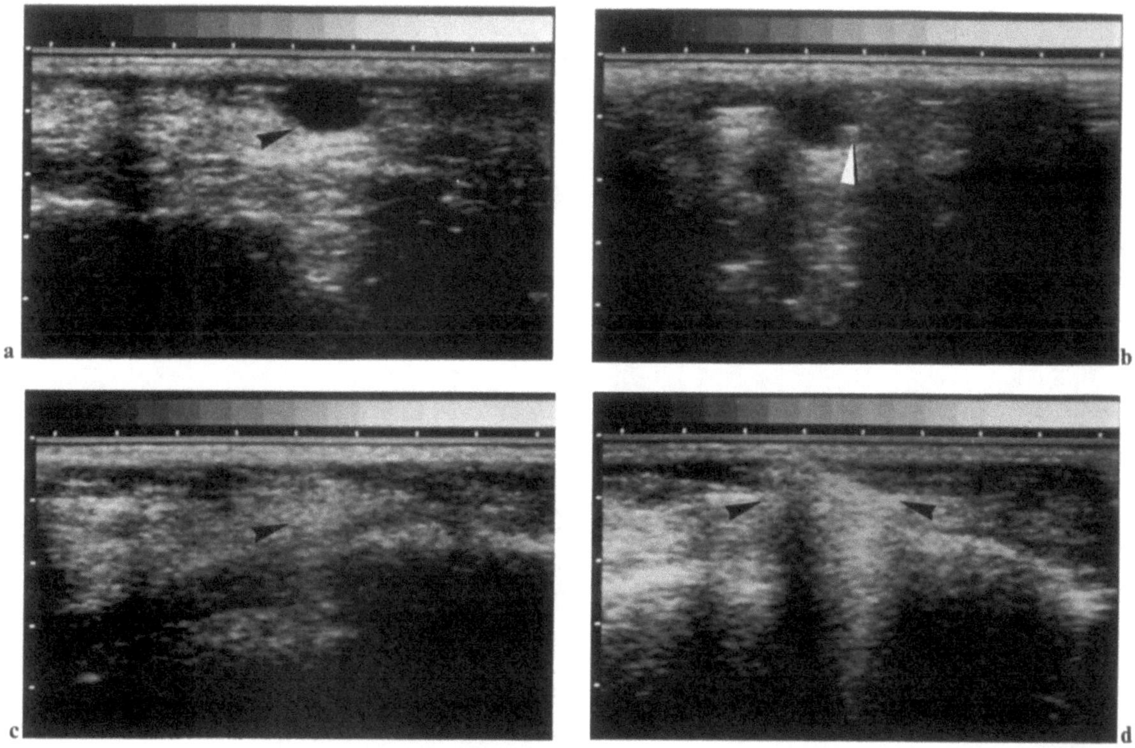

Fig. 5.19. **a** Cyst prior to aspiration. **b** Needle tip in the cyst interior. **c** Cyst is completely evacuated. **d** Appearance after air injection

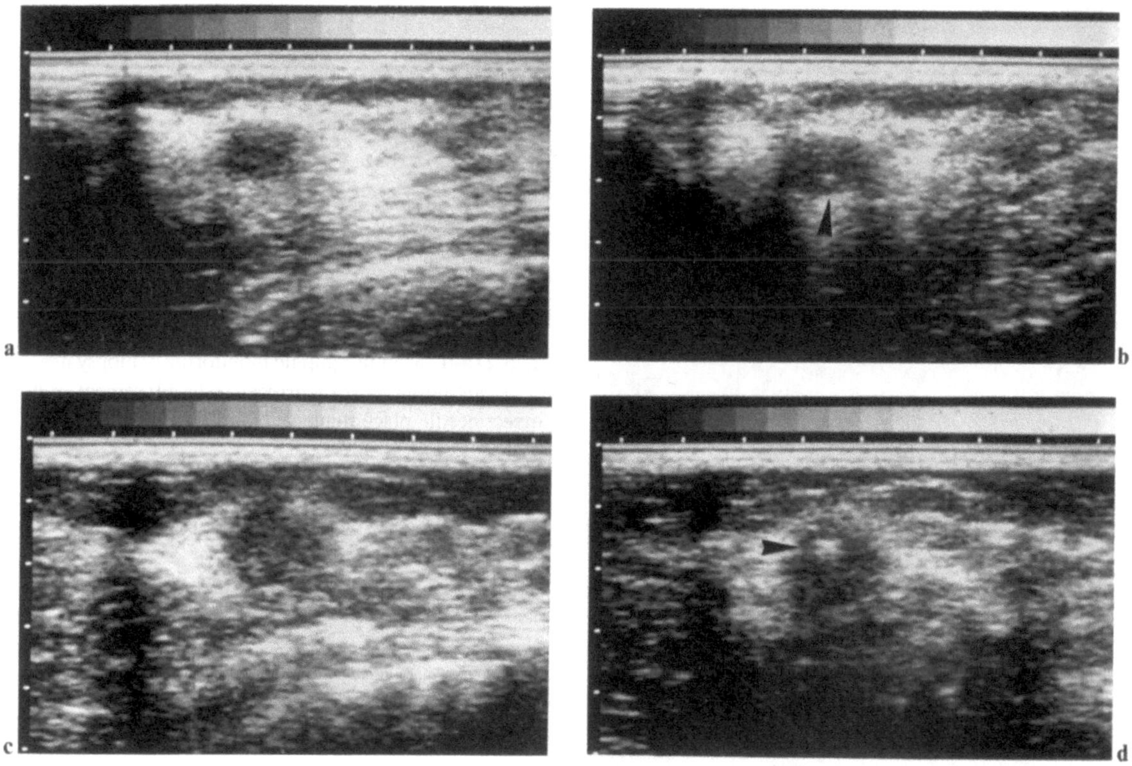

Fig. 5.20a-d. Echographic documentation of needle placement in solid masses. **a,b** Fibroadenoma. **c,d** Carcinoma

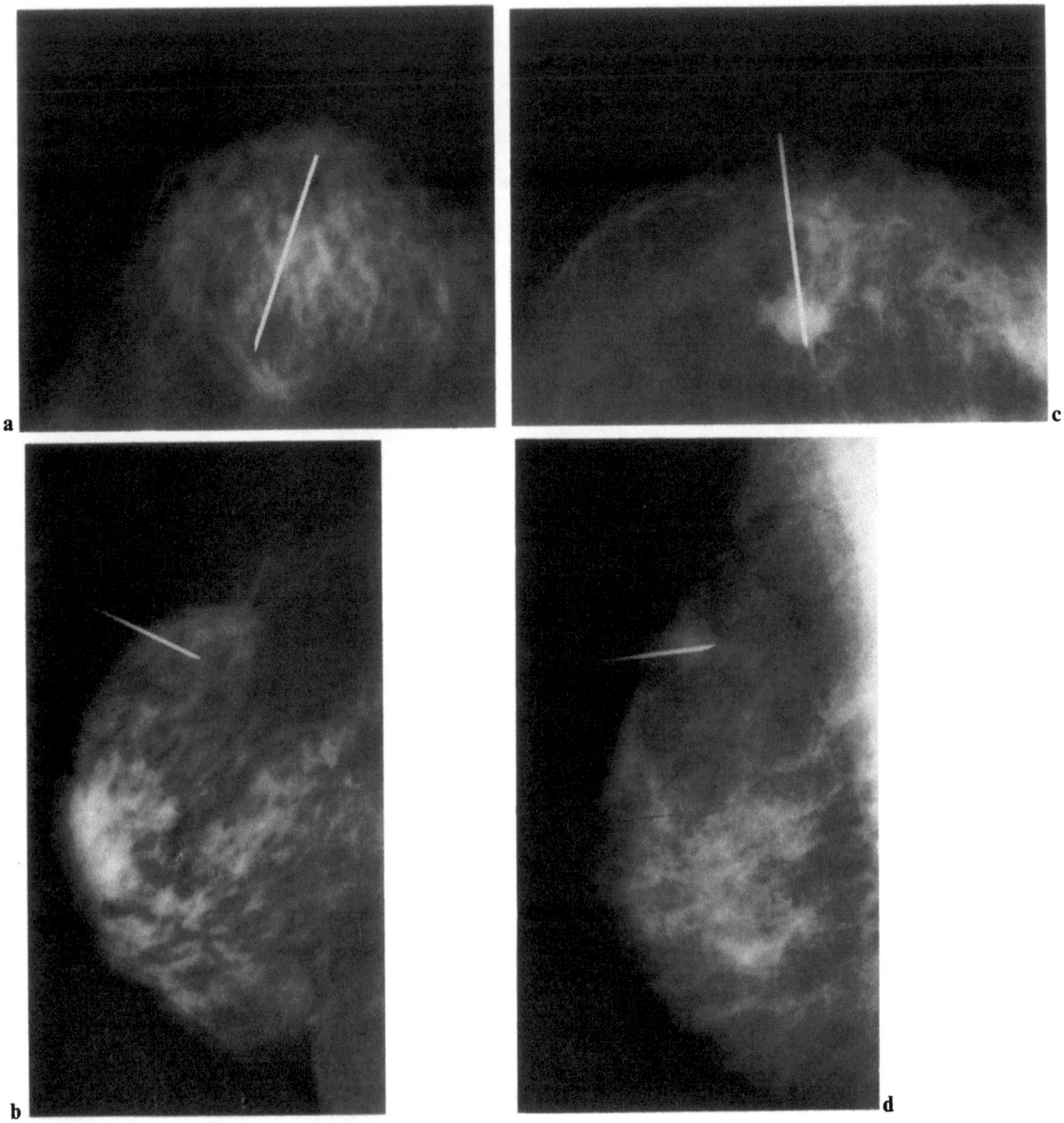

Fig. 5.21a-d. Mammographic monitoring of biopsy needle in carcinoma. **a,b** Incorrect needle placement. **c,d** Correct needle placement

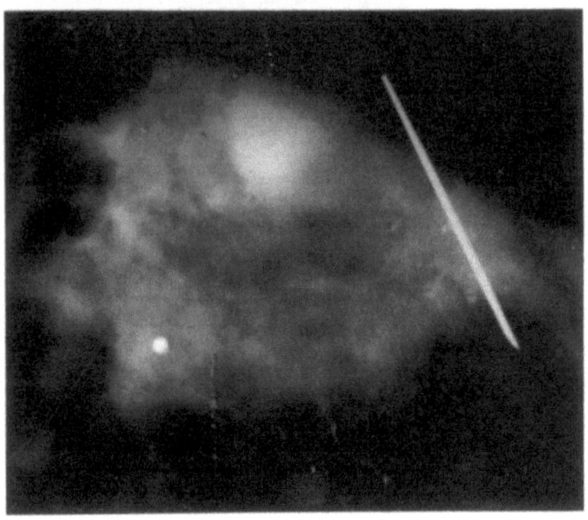

Fig. 5.22. Mammographic monitoring of biopsy needle in microcalcifications

Sonography Versus Pathohistology

Ultrasound established itself relatively quickly as the method of choice for the cystic/solid differentiation of masses. But what is its value in differentiating between benign and malignant breast lesions? One way to approach this question is by comparing the frequencies of benign mass and malignancy criteria for fibroadenomas and carcinomas (Table 5.11, 5.12). If we add together the corresponding criteria for an individual lesion in both categories and compare the sums, we can classify the result as suggestive of a benign mass ($\Sigma_b > \Sigma_m$), suggestive of malignancy ($\Sigma_b < \Sigma_m$), or indifferent ($\Sigma_b = \Sigma_m$) (Table 5.13). This method has an 87% accuracy rate in carcinomas and an 83% accuracy rate in fibroadenomas. In that regard our results agree roughly with those of other groups of workers. They demonstrate the relatively high accuracy of ultrasound in identifying preoperatively the nature of a focal lesion, even (and especially) in comparison with corresponding clinical and radiographic results (Table 5.14).

The sonographic assessment of tumor margins naturally becomes more difficult and less precise as the boundaries of the tumor become less well defined. In most cases it is possible only to delineate the hypoechoic core of the mass. Occasionally it is better to include the hyperechoic rim when measuring the diameter of the mass (Fig. 5.23). This "echogenic rim" (Teubner, 1985) can be seen very clearly on hand-held real-time scans; it is less apparent on static images and on immersion scans due to the absence of breast compression. Preoperative sonographic tumor measurement yields fairly accurate values for carcinomas with a pathohistologic diameter of 1 to 2 cm. There is a tendency to overestimate the sizes of smaller carcinomas, and to underestimate the sizes of tumors larger than 2 cm (Fig. 5.24).

Table 5.11. Ultrasound criteria for benign mass.

Criterion	Carcinomas N=200 (%)	Fibroadenomas N=80 (%)
Smooth margins	1	60
Halo	0	71
Lateral shadowing	0	45
Uniform distribution of internal echoes	21	82
Regular structure of internal echoes	10	68
Enhancement behind entire lesion	11	24
Enhancement on both planes of examination	7	13

Table 5.12. Ultrasound criteria for malignancy.

Criterion	Carcinomas N=200 (%)	Fibroadenomas N=80 (%)
Ill-defined margins	84	12
Broom-straw pattern (hyperechoic)	64	0
Fir-tree pattern (hypoechoic)	24	0
Nonuniform distribution of internal echoes	66	17
Irregular structure of internal echoes	71	12
Shadowing (central)	74	5
Shadowing on both planes of examination	56	5

Table 5.13. Accuracy of preoperative assessment of benign mass and malignancy using the method of criteria addition.

Accuracy[a]	Carcinomas (%)	Fibroadenomas (%)
$\Sigma_b > \Sigma_m$ = suggestive of benign mass	6	83
$\Sigma_b = \Sigma_m$ = indifferent	7	5
$\Sigma_b < \Sigma_m$ = suggestive of malignancy	87	12

[a] Σ_b = sum of benign mass criteria; Σ_m = sum of malignancy criteria.

Table 5.14. Accuracy rates in assessment of benign mass and malignancy.

Study	Correct preoperative classification as	
	Benign	Malignant
Clinical impression		
Kreuzer et al., 1973	77% (*n*=656)	57% (*n*=369)
Radiography		
Kreuzer et al., 1973	39% (*n*=656)	74% (*n*=369)
Wellern, 1978	45% (*n*=852)	62% (*n*=300)
De Gezelle et al., 1981		80% (*n*=51)
Fleischer et al., 1983	68% (*n*=25)	
Stosiek et al., 1983	75% (*n*=147)	82% (*n*=97)
Leucht et al., 1985	73% (*n*=78)	82% (*n*=197)
Total	60% (*n*=1758)	76% (*n*=1014)
Ultrasound		
Kobayashi, 1980	83% (*n*=938)	85% (*n*=1180)
De Gezelle et al., 1981		86% (*n*=51)
Cole-Beuglet et al., 1983	83% (*n*=52)	
Fleischer et al., 1983	68% (*n*=25)	
Kelly-Fry and Harper, 1983		95% (*n*=73)
Kessler et al., 1983		88% (*n*=94)
Stosiek et al., 1983	85% (*n*=147)	79% (*n*=97)
Egan and Egan, 1984	83% (*n*=69)	87% (*n*=107)
Leucht et al., 1985	71% (*n*=78)	91% (*n*=197)
Subtotal	81% (*n*=1309)	85% (*n*=1726)
Our results	83% (*n*=76)	87% (*n*=196)
Total	82% (*n*=1385)	86% (*n*=1922)

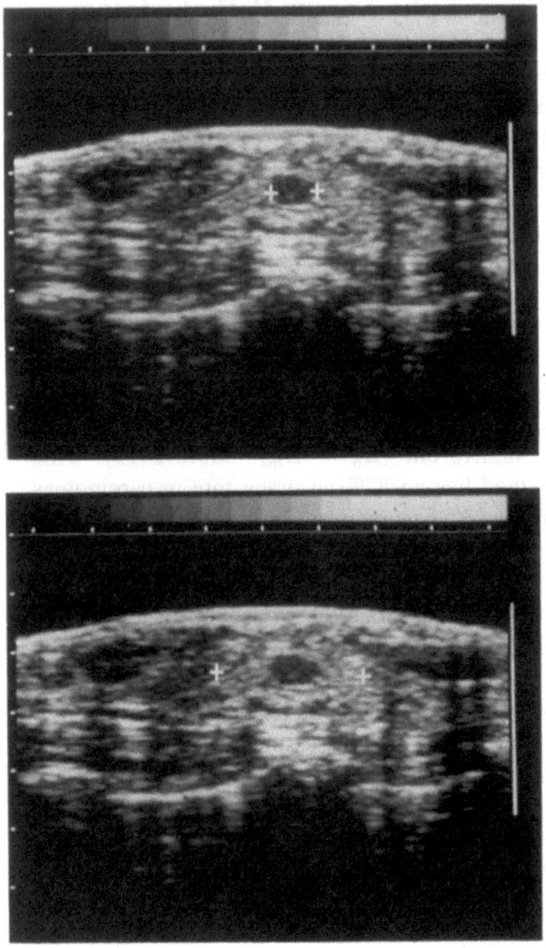

a

b

Fig. 5.23a,b. Measurement of (**a**) the hypoechoic core of the mass (8 mm) and (**b**) of the entire lesion, including the echogenic halo (25 mm), in a predominantly intraductal comedocarcinoma that measured 3×2.5 cm on pathohistologic examination

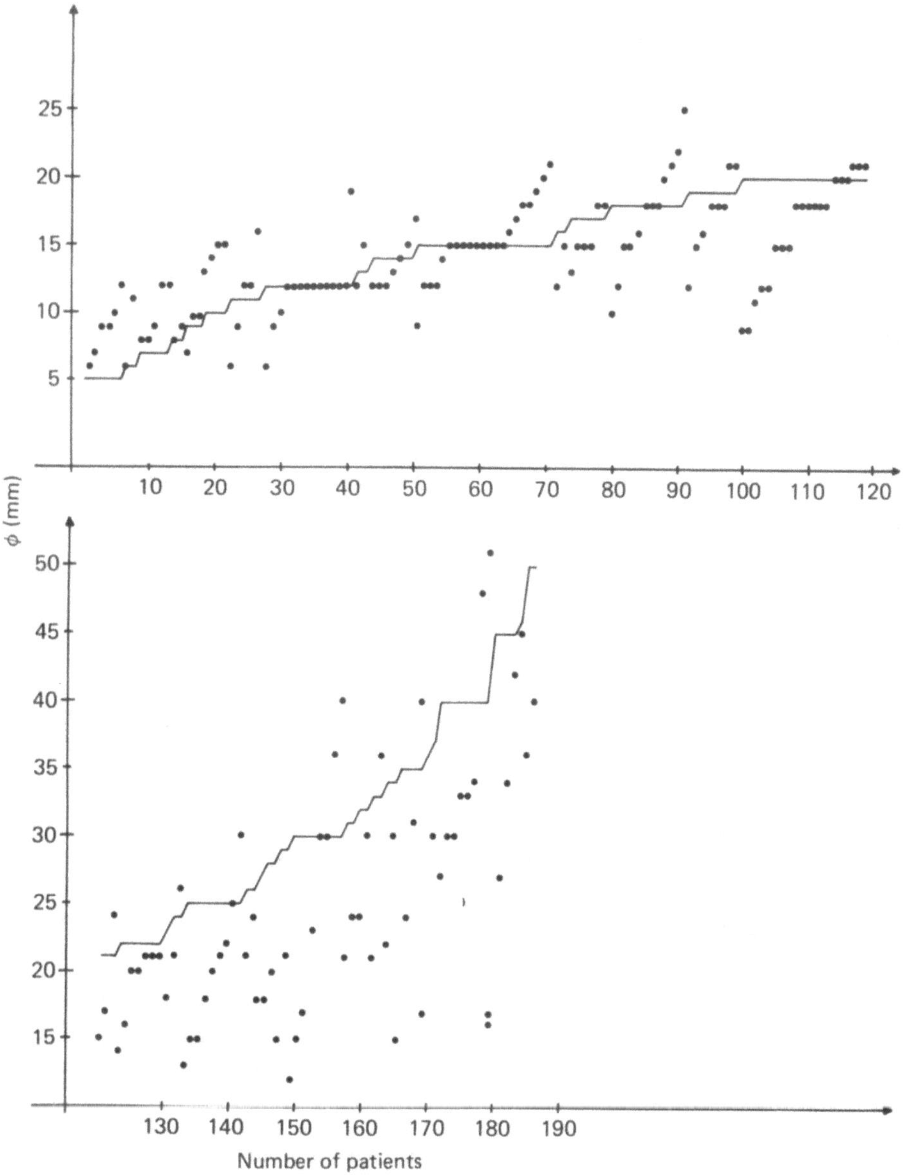

Fig. 5.24. Comparison of the largest measured diameters of 185 carcinomas in pathohistologic sections (solid line) and on sonograms (dots)

Bibliography

Abe, R., Kimura, M., Sato, T., Yoshida, K., Hariu, T., Kanno, H., Takahashi, K., Matoba, N., Kumagai, N. (1985). Trial of early detection of breast cancer by mass screening. *Cancer 56*:1479–1483.

Amalric, R., Spitalier, J.M., Levraud, J., Altschuler, C. (1972). Classification des images thermovisuelles des carcinomes mammaires. Lecture, International Breast Symposium, Strassburg, France.

Barth, V. (1977). *Atlas der Brustdrüsenerkrankungen*. Enke, Stuttgart, France.

Bastert, G., Nagel, G.A., Rauschecker, H., Sauer, R., Schauer, A. (1985). Basisempfehlungen zur Diagnostik, Therapie und Nachsorge beim Mammakarzinom. *Deutsches Ärzteblatt 82*:2258–2264.

Bogin, I.N., Shapiro, Shunaeva, Bogdanov, Poltoratskaia (1979). Combined use of thermography, bioecholocation and aspiration biopsy in the diagnosis of breast diseases. *Klinicheskaia Meditsina 57*:47–50.

Bolmgren, J., Jacobson, B., Nordenström, B. (1977). Stereotaxic instrument for needle biopsy of the mamma. *American Journal of Roentgenology 129*:121–125.

Breyer, B., Cepulić, E., Zunter, F. (1982). Ultrasonic mammography without specialized equipment: comparison with clinical examinations and X-rays. *Ultrasound in Medicine and Biology 8*:377–379.

Cole-Beuglet, C., Goldberg, B.B., Kurtz, A.B., Rubin, C.S., Patchefsky, A.S., Shaber, G.S. (1981). Ultrasound mammography: A comparison with radiographic mammography. *Radiology 139*:693–698.

Cole-Beuglet, C., Soriano, R.Z., Kurtz, A.B., Goldberg, B.B. (1983). Fibroadenoma of the breast: Sonomammography correlated with pathology in 122 patients. *American Journal of Roentgenology 140*:369–375.

Croll, J. (1985). Sonography in the Young Symptomatic Patient and in Some Confusing and Unusual Cases of Benign Disease. In Jellins, Kossoff, Croll (Eds.), *Proceedings of the 4th International Congress on the Ultrasonic Examination of the Breast*. Witton Press Pty. Ltd., Sydney, Australia, pp. 65–72.

DeGezelle, H., Vanpeperstraete, A., Defoort, P., Serreyn, R., Vandekerckhove, D. (1981). Comparison of breast tumours evaluated by ultrasound, mammography, and clinical investigation. *Archives of Gynecology 230*:219–223.

Duda, V. (1982). *Ultraschall-Mammographie: Das sonographische Erscheinungsbild anatomischer und pathologischer Strukturen der Mamma unter Anwendung eines Immersionsscanners*. Dissertation, University of Marburg, West Germany, pp. 98–108.

Egan, R.L., Egan, K.L. (1984). Detection of breast carcinoma: Comparison of automated water-path whole-breast sonography, mammography, and physical examination. *American Journal of Roentgenology 143*:493–497.

Egan, R.L., Egan, K.L. (1984). Automated water-path full-breast sonography: Correlation with histology of 176 solid lesions. *American Journal of Roentgenology 143*:499–507.

Elling, D., Abet, L., Lenke, S., Kobs, K. (1982). Erste Erfahrungen mit der kombinierten ultrasonographischen und röntgenmammographischen Diagnostik von cystischen Mammatumoren. *Zentralblatt der Gynäkology 104*:1234–1239.

Eulenburg, R., Hackelöer, B.J., Lauth, G., Hüneke, B., Duda, V., Buchholz, R. (1981). Ultraschall-Mammografie: Spezielle Einsatzbereiche. *Geburtshilfe Frauenheilkunde 41*:169–172.

Feig, S.A. (1985). Benefits, risks, and costs of mammographic screening. In Mardaga (Ed.), *Proceedings of the International Symposium of Senology*, 7–9 Nov. 1985, Liège, Belgium, pp. 123–133.

Fields, S.I. (1980). Ultrasound mammographic-histopathologic correlation. *Ultrasonic Imaging 2*:150–161.

Fleischer, A.C., Muhletaler, C.A., Reynolds, V.H., Machin, J.E., Thieme, G.A., Bundy, A.L., Winfield, A.C., James, Jr., A.E. (1983). Palpable breast masses: Evaluation by high frequency, hand-held real-time sonography and xeromammography. *Radiology 148*:813–817.

Frazier, T.G., Cole-Beuglet, C., Kurtz, A.B., Goldberg, B.B., Ryan, S.M. (1982). Further evaluation by ultrasound of mammographically determined breast dysplasia. *Journal of Surgical Oncology 19*:69–70.

Friedrich, M. (1978). Neue Entwicklungstendenzen der Mammographie-Technik: Die Rastermammographie. *Fortschritte der Röntgenstrahlen 128*:207–222.

Friedrich, M. (1981). Neue technische Entwicklungen der Röntgen- und Ultraschalluntersuchung der Mamma. *Röntgenpraxis 34*:181–195.

Frischbier, H.J. (1985). Screening program with mammography in Hamburg. In Mardaga (Ed.), *Proceedings of the International Symposium of Senology*, 7–9 Nov. 1985, Liège, Belgium, pp. 99–105.

Frischbier, H.J., Lohbeck, H.V. (1977). *Frühdiagnostik des Mamma-Karzinoms*. Thieme, Stuttgart, France.

Gautherie, M. (1983). Thermobiological assessment of benign and malignant breast diseases. *American Journal of Obstetrics and Gynecology 147*:861–870.

Gautherie, M., Gros, Ch.M. (1980). Breast thermography and cancer risk prediction. *Cancer 45*:51–56.

Gautherie, M., Kotewicz, A., Gueblez, P. (1984). Accurate and objective evaluation of breast thermograms: Basic principles and new advances with special reference to an improved computer assisted scoring system. In Gautherie, Albert, Keith (Eds.), *Thermal Assessment of Breast Health*. MTP Press, London, pp. 74–97.

Good, M.S., Rose, J.L., Goldberg, B.B. (1982). Application of pattern recognition techniques to breast cancer detection: Ultrasonic analysis of 100 pathologically confirmed tissue areas. *Ultrasonic Imaging 4*:378-396.

Gros, Ch., Dale, G., Gairard, B., Gautherie, M. (1975). Corrélations échothermographiques mammaires. *Nucléaire 56*:481-486.

Harper, A.P., Jackson, V.P., Bies, J., Ransburg, R., Kelly-Fry, E., Noe, J.S. (1982). A preliminary analysis of the ultrasound imaging characteristics of malignant breast masses as compared with X-ray mammographic appearances and the gross and microscopic pathology. *Ultrasound in Medicine and Biology 8*:365-368.

Harper, A.P., Kelly-Fry, E. (1978). Combined use of mammography and ultrasound visualization using a laboratory-modified commercial breast scanner to improve differential diagnosis. In *Proceedings of the 23rd Annual Meeting of AIUM* p. 131. Oct. 19-23, 1978, San Diego.

Harper, A.P., Kelly-Fry, E. (1980). Ultrasound visualization of the breast in symptomatic patients. *Radiology 137*:465-469.

Harper, A.P., Kelly-Fry, E. (1981). Ultrasound breast imaging—the method of choice for examining the young patient. *Ultrasound in Medicine and Biology 7*:231-237.

Hoeffken, W., Lanyi, M. (1973). *Röntgenuntersuchung der Brust*. Thieme, Stuttgart, France.

Hüneke, B. (1982). *Ultraschallmammographie: Stellenwert und Bedeutung der Methode im Vergleich mit Röntgenmammographie, Thermographie und Feinnadelbiopsie*. Dissertation, University of Marburg, West Germany, pp. 1-201.

Igl, W., Lohe, K., Eiermann, W., Bassermann, R., Lissner, J. (1980). Sonographische carcinomdiagnostik der weiblichen Brust im Vergleich zur Mammographie. *Tumordiagnostik 5*:247-253.

Jellins, J., Reeve, T.S. (1978). Breast echography compared with xerography. *Ultrasound in Medicine 4*:313-318.

Kasumi, F. (1985). Physiological patterns and benign disease diagnosis. In Jellins, Kossoff, Croll (Eds.), *Proceedings of the 4th International Congress on the Ultrasonic Examination of the Breast*. Witton Press Pty. Ltd., Sydney, Australia, pp. 57-63.

Kessler M., Igl W., Bassermann, R., et al. (1983b). Ergebnisse von Mammographie und Mammasonographie mit manuellem und automatisiertem Scanvorgang. In Otto/Jann (Ed.), *Ultraschalldiagnostik '82*; Thieme, Stuttgart-New York, pp. 362-365.

Kessler, M., Igl, W., Valena, D., Bassermann, R., Bohmert, D.H., Eiermann, W., Lohe, K.J. (1983a). Vergleich von Mammographie und Mamma-Sonographie mit verschiedenen Gerätetypen. Aussagekraft und Stellenwert. Lecture, Gemeinsame Jahrestagung 1983 der Hessischen Gesellschaft für Medizinische Strahlenkunde, der Vereinigung Südwestdeutscher Radiologen und Nuklearmediziner und der Bayerischen Röntgengesellschaft, Darmstadt, West Germany.

Kindermann, G. (1985). Diagnostic value of galactography in the detection of breast cancer. In Zander and Baltzer (Eds.), *Early Breast Cancer*. Springer-Verlag, Berlin, Heidelberg, New York, pp 137-139.

Kobayashi, T. (1979). Diagnostic ultrasound in breast cancer: Analysis of retrotumorous echo patterns correlated with sonic attenuation by cancerous connective tissue. *Journal of Clinical Ultrasound 7*:471-479.

Kobayashi, T. (1980). *Gray Scale Echography for Breast Cancer*. Hitachi Medical Corporation, Tokyo, Japan, No. 639.

Kobayashi, T. (1983). Screening of breast cancer by echography in cancer detection center. Abstract, *3rd International Congress on the Ultrasonic Examination of the Breast* (Vol. 63). Tokyo, 10-12 June 1983.

Kopans, D.B., Meyer, J.E., Lindfors, K.K., Bucchianeri, S.S. (1984). Breast sonography to guide cyst aspiration and wire localization of occult solid lesions. *American Journal of Roentgenology 143*:489-492.

Kreuzer, G., Boquoi, E., Meyer, R.D. (1973). Die diagnostik gut- und bösartiger mammatumoren. *Deutsche Medizinische Wochenschrift 98*:691-698.

Laing, F.C., Jeffrey, R.B., Minagi, H. (1984). Ultrasound localization of occult breast lesions. *Radiology 151*:795-796.

Lambie, R.W., Hodgden, D., Herman, E.M., Kopperman, M. (1983a). Sonomammographic detection of lobular carcinoma not demonstrated on xeromammography. *Journal of Clinical Ultrasound 11*:495-497.

Lambie, R.W., Hodgden, D., Herman, E.M., Kopperman, M. (1983b). Sonomammographic manifestations of mammographically detectable breast microcalcifications. *Journal of Ultrasound in Medicine 2*:509-514.

Lanyi, M. (1985). Morphological analysis of microcalcifications. In Zander and Baltzer (Eds.), *Early Breast Cancer*. Springer-Verlag, Berlin, Heidelberg, New York, pp. 113-135.

Lapayowker, M.S., Revesz, G. (1980). Thermography and ultrasound in detection and diagnosis of breast cancer. *Cancer 46*:933-938.

Lauth, G., Duda, V., Hackelöer, B.J. (1985). Ultrasound mammography: Possibilities and limitations in the detection of early breast cancer. In Zander and Baltzer (Eds.), *Early Breast Cancer*. Springer-Verlag, Berlin, Heidelberg, New York, pp. 174-178.

Lauth, G., Eulenburg, R. (1986). *Angewandte Thermologie* (Vol. 3). *Thermographie der weiblichen Brust*. Edition Medizin, VCH Verlagsgesellschaft, Weinheim, West Germany.

Lauth, G., Eulenburg, R., Hackelöer, B.J., Duda, V., Hüneke, B., Buchholz, R. (1982). Röntgen-Mammographie und Sonographie der Brust–Ein Vergleich. *Röntgen-Blätter 35*:359–363.

Lauth, G., Mühlberger, G. (1976). In CAWO GmbH (Ed.), *Atlas der Plattenthermographie*. Staudt Druck KG, Geisenfeld, West Germany.

Leucht, W., Rabe, D., Müller, A., von Fournier, D., Humbert, K.D., Schmidt, W. (1985). Verbesserung der präoperativen Abklärung von palpablen, nichtzystischen Prozessen der Mamma durch die Echomammographie. *Ultraschall 6*:15–25.

Lundgren, B. (1979). Population screening for breast cancer by single view mammography in a geographic region of Sweden. JNCL *62*:1373–1379.

Mustacchi, G., Milani, S., Forlivesi, L., Risaliti, A. (1980). Integrated mammillary diagnostic experience: Telethermography, mammography, echography, cytology. *European Journal of Gynaecological Oncology 1*:185–187.

Nitschke, S., Lauth, G., Hackelöer, B.J. (1978). A new ultrasonographic method for the diagnosis and puncture of mammarian cysts. Lecture, 3rd European Congress on Ultrasonics in Medicine, Bologne, Italy.

Nordenström, B., Zajicek, J. (1977). Stereotaxic needle biopsy and preoperative indication of non-palpable mammary lesions. *Acta Cytologica 21*:350–351.

Novak, D. (1983). Indications for and comparative diagnostic value of combined ultrasound and X-ray mammography. *European Journal of Radiology 3*, Suppl. 1:299–302.

Ossoinig K., Kaiser, P., Kolb, R., Lechner, G. (1971). Echographische und röntgenologische Befunde bei Erkrankungen der Mamma. *Ultrasonographia Medica III*:127–138.

Otto, R., Engeler, V. (1980). Die ultraschallgezielte Punktion von Mammazysten. Lecture, 1st World Congress on Senology, Hamburg.

Pirschel, J. (1983). Mammasonographie im real-time Immersionsverfahren–sonographische, mammographische und histologische Befunde. Habilitationsschrift, University of Tübingen; West Germany, pp. 1–191.

Resta, P., Nardelli, G.B., Ambrosini, A., Becagli, L., D'Antona, N. (1980). Echography and Mammography in Breast Neoplasias. *European Journal of Gynaecological Oncology 1*:181–184.

Rosner, D. (1981). Ultrasonography in Diagnosis and Management of Palpable Breast Masses. *New York State Journal of Medicine 81*:1066–1072.

Sickles, E.A., Filly, R.A., Callen, P.W. (1983). Breast cancer detection with sonography and mammography: Comparison using state-of-the-art equipment. *American Journal of Roentgenology 140*:843–845.

Skaane, P., Bautz, W., Metzger, H. (1985). Die umschriebene und diffuse Hautverdickung (peau d'orange) der weiblichen Brustdrüse. *RöFo 143*:212–219.

Stosiek, U., Breitbach, G.P., Linder, R. (1983). Kombinierte präoperative Diagnostik von Mammatumoren. *Tumordiagnostik & Therapie 4*:175–178.

Teiidor, H.S., Kazam, E. (1977). Combined mammographic-sonographic evaluation of breast masses. *American Journal of Roentgenology 128*: 409–417.

Teubner, J. (1985). Der echodichte Randsaum: Ein wichtiges Tumorkriterium mit hoher diagnostischer Wertigkeit bei der Mammasonographie. In G. Judmaier, H. Tsonienhold, A. Kratochwil (Eds.), *Ultraschalldiagnostik 84*. G. Thieme, Stuttgart-New York, pp. 367–368.

Thiel, C., Schweikhart, G. (1982). Ultraschallmammographie: Ihre Bedeutung im Rahmen einer integrierten Mammadiagnostik. *RöFo 137*:1–12.

Tricoire, J. (1970). La thermographie en plaque. Technique nouvelle d'utilization des cristeaux liquides. *Presse Medicale 78*:2481.

Tricoire, J. (1973). Das diagnostische Verfahren der Plattenthermographie unter besonderer Berücksichtigung der Untersuchung der weiblichen Brust. *Das ärztliche Gespräch*. Troponwerke, Cologne, pp. 16–26.

Wagai, T., Tsutsumi, M. (1983). Screening trial of breast cancer by echography. Abstract, 3rd International Congress of Ultrasonic Examination of the Breast (Vol. 58), Tokyo, 10–12 June 1983.

Wellern, G. (1978). *Die Treffsicherheit der Mammographie und die Wertigkeit des mammographischen Einzelsymptoms*. Dissertation, University of Marburg, West Germany.

Wolf, G., Hohenberg, G. (1984). Mammographisches und sonographisches Erscheinungsbild traumatischer Veränderungen der weiblichen Brust. *RöFo 141*: 204–208.

Zander, J., Baltzer, J. (1985). *Early Breast Cancer*. Springer-Verlag, Berlin, Heidelberg, New York.

6
Evolution and Status of Breast Sonography: Instrumentation and User Requirements

The technical evolution of ultrasound mammography is outlined in Table 6.1. To date there has been little experience with the latest generation of instruments for computed sonography, although I mentioned these systems briefly in my discussion of microcalcifications (Chap. 5.3).

Hand-held compound scanners are rarely used nowadays and offer no advantages over other instrument types. Automated immersion scanners are still the only systems that provide an uncompressed whole-breast image, although their application is relatively limited. These instruments have been of major importance in a didactic sense, however, and they have performed a pace-setting role. Disadvantages are their high cost and the substantial amount of time needed to conduct an examination. While only a few of these instruments are operational in Europe, they have found considerably broader use in the United States and Australia for reasons relating to history and personnel.

In the United States and Japan, the most commonly used dedicated ultrasound breast scanner is probably a supine scanner. These scanners have been commercially available and routinely used in Japan for well over ten years. An automated unit originally developed at Indiana University Medical School is presently being used in at least 150 United States medical centers or private breast clinics.

Automated scanners are now experiencing a comeback. As far as we are concerned, in the near future a well-run breast center will include both hand-held and automated ultrasound mammography units. Real-time systems are very helpful in diagnosis but because of the missing standard examination planes there is a difficulty in orientation. With their sharply focused transducers, automated systems can provide better resolution.

Our approach is to have the patient first in a supine position and to scan the breast with an automated system, using the best method of orientation and resolution. Once the area of interest has been defined, the patient is turned to a prone position. The breast area under consideration is then rescanned with a hand-held unit. The prone position not only allows performance of necessary palpations but also allows forms of intervention, such as fine needle biopsy. All such interventions may be immediately carried out under ultrasound guidance.

Table 6.1. History of the development of ultrasound mammography.

Authors	Remarks
Wild and Reid, 1952	Echoscope, A scan, 15 MHz, 21 cases, first B scans
Howry et al., 1954	Somascope, B scan, 2 MHz, experiments on surgical specimens
Kickuchi et al., 1957	A + B scan, 5–10 MHz, water bag
Wells and Evans, 1968	Water tank scanner, sector B scan, 2 MHz, examination in prone position
Kelly-Fry, 1968	Breast tissue characterization by computer controlled, multiple focus, 3 MHz system
Damascelli et al., 1970	Diasonograph, compound-contact B scan, 2.5–5 MHz, 38 cases
Jellins et al., 1971	Ultrasonic echoscope, water tank scanner, 2 MHz
Kelly-Fry et al., 1972	Benign and Malignant Echo Patterns by computerized, automated 3.0, 2.2, 1.7 MHz system
Kossoff and Garrett, 1972	Film echograph = gray-scale imaging
Kossoff et al., 1973	Measured velocity of sound propagation in breast tissue
Wagai, 1974	Arc scanner, 5 MHz, gray-scale imaging, water bag, supine position
Kobayashi, 1974	Sonolayergraph, 2–6 MHz, criteria for benign mass and malignancy, sensitivity-graded method
Kossoff et al., 1975	Octoson (automated immersion scanner), eight 3-MHz transducers
Cole-Beuglet and Beique, 1975	Vidoson, 2.5 MHz Bronson Turner, 7–8 MHz, real-time, 180 cases
Gros et al., 1975	A + B scan, 6–8.5 MHz, criteria for benign mass and malignancy
Calderon et al., 1976	Measurement of attenuation in normal, benign, and malignant breast tissues
Wagai and Tsutsumi, 1977	Screening examinations using technique of 1974 (see above)
Kobayashi et al., 1977	Expanded echogram = electronic image sector enlargement
Baum, 1977	Immersion scanner, 2.25 MHz, examination in sitting position
Kelly-Fry et al., 1979	Fast Fourier Transform techniques for attenuation characteristics of malignant breast tumors
Rubin et al., 1979	Octoson, 3 MHz, parenchymal patterns
Bielke et al., 1980	Combison 100, 3.5 MHz, special water-path transducer system, examination in sitting position
Harper and Kelly-Fry, 1980	Automated, sharply focused 3.7 MHz system, supine position, compressed breast
Carson et al., 1981	Transmission ultrasound, 3.5 MHz, coronal planes
Foster et al., 1983	Annular array scanner, conical transducer, 4 MHz
Bloomberg et al., 1984	Linear array scanner, 5 MHz, real-time characteristics of the breast
Hackelöer et al., 1986	Acuson, 5 MHz, linear array, computed sonography

Table 6.2. Recommendations on the use of breast sonography.

Instrument requirements for	Indications for use	Physician Requirements
1. Real-time linear scanner should meet these criteria: a) Operating frequency ≥ 5 MHz b) At least 5 cm width and depth of image field c) Electronic focusing over a depth range of 0.5–5 cm with direct transducer coupling; water-path coupling requires extending depth range by length of water path	Mammography should always precede breast sonography, except in women under age 30 with a palable breast mass, where sonography may be used as primary examination for cyst detection. Sonography may be used in women with proven gross cystic disease to confirm cystic nature of new palpable mass found between regular follow-up mammograms.	1. Practice sonography according to established techniques of breast ultrasound
2. Mechanical real-time scanners must guarantee image quality consistent with criteria in 1, regardless of operating frequency.	At present breast sonography is considered only as adjunct to mammography, and indicated only when suspicious mammographic fingind cannot be adequately investigated with X-ray techniques. Mammographically detected microcalcifications are not considered indication for breast ultrasound	2. Clinical, mammographic, and sonographic experience in at least 400 breast examinations performed and evaluated under direction of specialist during at least 4 months' full-time training or 2 years' part-time training. Certification of specialized knowledge of breast sonography by a board or committee is recommended.
3. Instruments with hand-held transducers and slow image buildup (compound scanners): minimum transducer frequency is 5 MHz. Small transducer face (6 mm) is needed for contact scans. Water-path scans require larger transducer face, depending on path length, with corresponding focal adjustment.		
4. Instruments that operate by different principles, such as immersion scanners, should satisfy image quality requirements as defined in 1.		

At the present time in Europe there is a definite preference for the use of real-time linear scanners in breast examinations. Coupling paths are used as required and are advantageous in some situations. The optimum transducer frequency is 5 MHz. Experiments using higher frequencies showed no advantages. Based on these findings, guidelines for breast ultrasound were developed by the German Institute for Ultrasound in Medicine (DEGUM) and the German Institute for Breast Study (Table 6.2).

Lower frequencies allow for examination of the nipple-areolar "shadow" area but higher frequencies, 7.5 to 10 MHz, permit detection of smaller lesions. For these reasons, the Kelly-Fry multiple frequency transducer was developed. We think it is essential to realize that frequency per se is not the only parameter important in diagnosis. It is quite possible, for example, to have a high frequency system with extremely poor resolution and a relatively low frequency system with resolution that may be better than that of some higher frequency systems (Kelly-Fry and Harper, 1983).

The capabilities of almost all commercially available instruments in given price ranges are comparable as far as image quality is concerned (Figs. 6.1-6.4). The price factor is important, since one would not expect the same performance from a compact as from a luxury sports car! The most modern instruments that feature fully computer-controlled signal and image processing, priced at about $100,000*, are priced well above the general range, as are the automated scanners, which range from about $70,000 to $200,000*. Serviceable real-time scanners can be purchased for $15,000 to $80,000. Before selecting an ultrasound instrument, it is important for the purchaser to assess personal capabilities and expectations. Quality requirements recommended by the Association of German Health Service Physicians are listed in Table 6.3 and may be considered to represent the minimum. One might say that a high instrument standard has already been reached today, but that future developments will raise the level of expectations even higher. The most pressing concern, however, is to improve the often very low quality standard of the professionals who conduct and interpret ultrasound examinations.

*These prices are projections and subject to fluctuation.

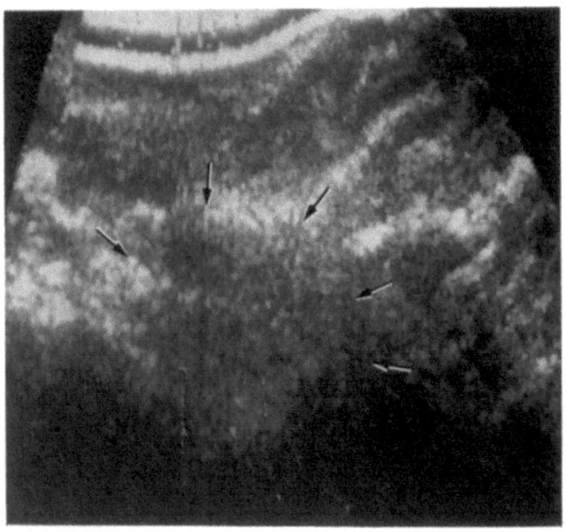

Fig. 6.1-6.4. Appearance of breast carcinoma on different ultrasound imaging systems

Fig. 6.1. Compound scan, 5 MHz

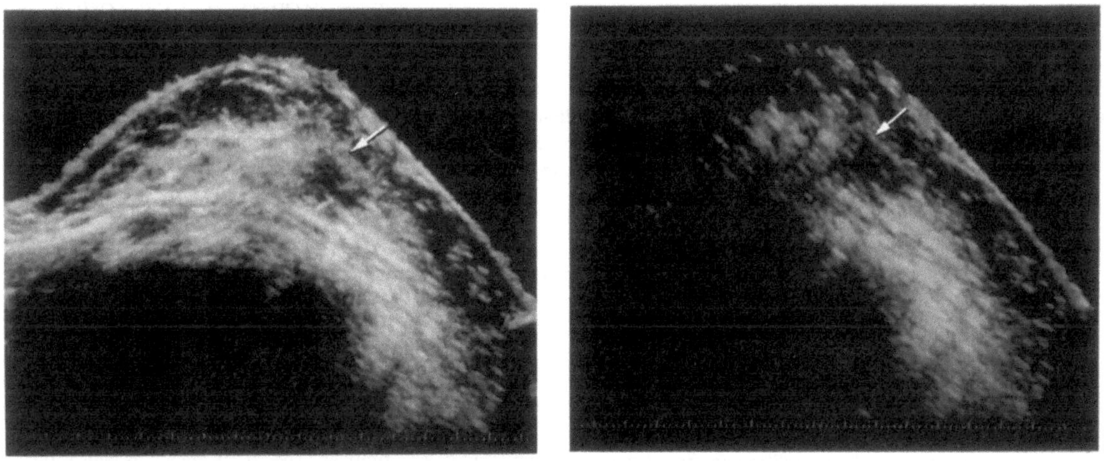

a b

Fig. 6.2a,b. Immersion scan. **a** Compound display, 4 transducers, 3 MHz. **b** Single scan, 1 transducer, 3 MHz

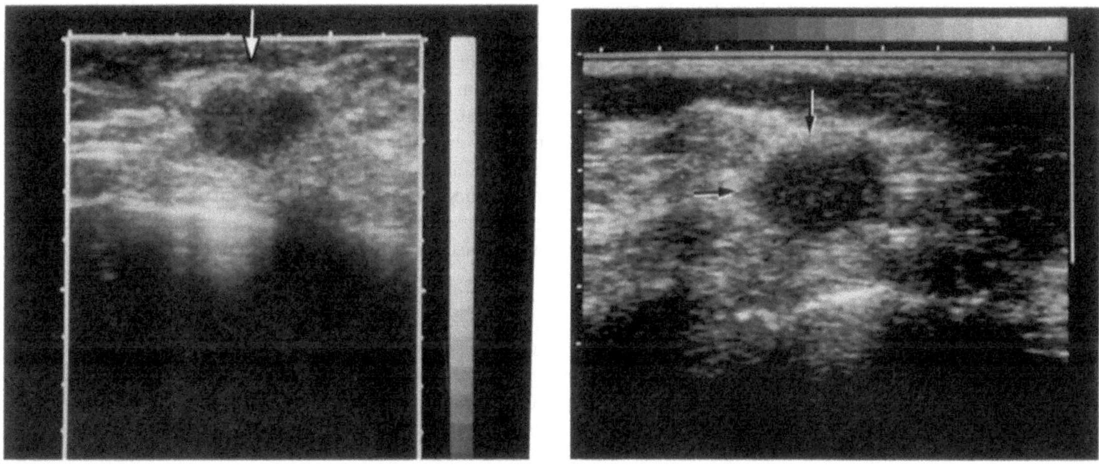

a b

Fig. 6.3a,b. Real-time scan. **a** 4–6 MHz without water path. **b** 5 MHz without water path

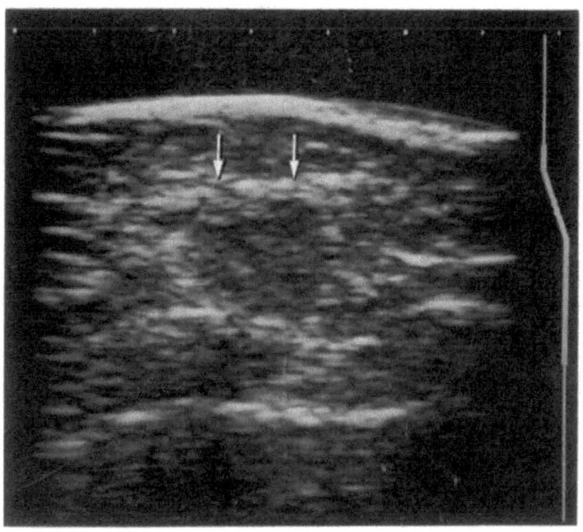

Fig. 6.4. Real-time scan, 5 MHz with water path

Policy Statement–on sonography for the detection and diagnosis of breast disease/ACR–The American College of Radiology, Chicago, IL 60606

Introduction

Ultrasound has been under investigation as a breast imaging modality for the past 30 years. The recent development of automated water-path scanning has allowed a more reliable evaluation of the entire breast. Commercially available breast sonography units differ in design and, therefore, scanning protocols and interpretive criteria are somewhat different.

Potential clinical indications for breast sonography

1. Evaluation of the symptomatic patient

The most important clinical role of breast sonography is to distinguish cysts from solid masses. Accuracy rates of 96–100 per cent are reported for sonography, exceeding those of mammography and physical examination. For palpable masses, any hand-held ultrasound unit having a transducer *frequency* of no lower than 5 MHz is accurate in identifying simple cysts, thereby averting unnecessary biopsies. The alternative technique of needle aspiration is diagnostic and may be faster and less expensive than ultrasound and usually is therapeutic for those masses that are cysts. Thus the greatest usefulness of sonography is when cyst-solid differentiations are needed for nonpalpable masses for which aspiration is impractical. These circumstances apply when noncalcified masses of indeterminate etiology are detected by mammography.

Breast sonography can also be utilitized for breast cancer detection, but its sensitivity and specificity are not as high as they are for cyst diagnosis. Sonographic differentiation of benign from malignant solid masses is not sufficiently reliable to direct clinical decisions, and sonographically solid masses must be considered potentially malignant, a situation that creates an unacceptably large number of false-positive diagnoses. Ultrasound is most helpful in the evaluation of uniformly dense breasts in which noncalcified cancers may go undetected by mammography. Most cancers that are identified by sonography also are palpable, indicating that the diagnostic contribution of sonography is limited. Futhermore, sonography is relatively ineffective in detecting carcinomas less than 1 cm in size, and the vast majority of cancers detected only as clustered calcifications by mammography are not imaged by ultrasound. Cancers are also difficult to detect sonographically in the fatty breast, for the hypoechoic pattern of most malignancies is similar to that of normal fat.

Because of these limitations, sonongraphy functions successfully only as an adjunct to mammography and physical examination. Its primary area of clinical usefulness is in making cyst-solid differentiations, particularly for nonpalpable mammographically-indeterminate masses. Sonography may prove useful in imaging palpable masses not detected by mammography, but needle aspiration usually proves sufficient in this clinical setting. One area in which breast ultrasound has been proposed as the initial imaging procedure is for women under age 30 in whom it is clinically important to establish or exclude the diagnosis of breast cysts. Further definition of this potential role is necessary.

2. Screening

The purpose of breast cancer screening is to detect clinically occult lesions. Breast sonography is currently limited in this regard by its inability to detect most malignancies presenting mammographically as clustered calcifications and by its difficulty in detecting cancers smaller than 1 cm in size. Because of these deficiencies, breast sonography should not be used as a screening modality.

Conclusions

1. Breast ultrasound is extremely accurate in distinguishing cysts from solid masses. Either aspiration or sonography should be performed prior to biopsy of ambiguous breast lesions to avert surgery of benign cysts.
2. Breast sonography does not reliably distinguish benign from malignant solid masses, fails to detect most cancers smaller than 1 cm in size, and almost never images cancers that present mammographically as clustered calcifications.

   Sonography should not be used for breast cancer screening or as the sole imaging modality in women with breast signs or symptoms suggesting the possibility of cancer.
3. Although breast sonography occasionally will provide clinically relevant information when used as an adjunct to physical examination and mammography, the additional cost of this examination precludes its routine use. Still undefined are specific clinical situations for which an additional sonographic examination is cost effective, but the most promising application appears to be the evaluation of questionably palpable masses in dense breasts where mammography shows no abnormality.
4. Further studies are necessary to define more precisely areas of clinical application for breast sonography, but until technological improvements permit a substantial increase in the accuracy of diagnosing nonpalpable carcinomas, the role of sonography will be limited primarily to making cyst-solid differentiations.

This policy statement is one of an occasional series reprinted by the American College of Radiology.
This formal statement of ACR policy was adopted by the Council on September 19, 1984.
Reprinted with permission from The American College of Radiology, Reston, Virginia, 1984.

Table 6.3. Example of guidelines for ultrasound examinations from Association of German Health Service Physicians, September 25, 1985.

Prerequisites

Diagnostic ultrasound of breast

At least 1 year's practical experience in general breast diagnosis (palpation, mammography, thermography, fine-needle biopsy) and examination of at least 200 patients in areas of surgery, radiology or gynecology

Instrument guidelines

Instrument safety: Instrument must meet appropriate specifications concerning use of high-frequency electronic equipment.

Biologic safety: Spatial-peak and time-average intensity of the ultrasound must conform to levels appropriate for application class. All instruments must have internal or external means for monitoring of essential system parameters. Following minimum requirements pertain to specific application classes.

Table 6.4.

Application class	Minimum apparatus	Minimum technical requirements for apparatus used
Breast diagnosis	Manual B-mode instrument for cross-sectional imaging	B-mode display utilizing image storage unit (analog or digital) with at least 16 amplitude levels (gray levels) manual scanning with transducer that can be freely moved on scan plane of interest; geometric error no greater than 5 mm, measured on suitable test object. Use of small-face (6 mm) contact transducer; image documentation with scale information; adjustable, calibrated transmitter output and/or receiver gain, and adjustable time gain compensation; readout on signal processing mode, where applicable; minimum ultrasound frequency (mean value) 5 MHz
	Or: Automated B-mode instrument for cross-sectional imaging (mechanical or electronic)	B-mode display, direct or using an image storage unit (analog or digital) with at least 16 amplitude levels (gray levels); geometric error no more than ±3% of test distance (error of 1 mm is permissible), measured on a suitable test object; image documentation with scale information; adjustable, calibrated transmitter output and/or receiver gain, and adjustable TGC; readout on signal processing mode, where applicable; minimum ultrasound frequency (mean value) 5 MHz, best resolution in region from 0.5–5 cm (focal region), image width and depth at least 5 cm past skin surface

Bibliography

Baum, G. (1977). Ultrasound mammography. *Radiology 122*:199–205.

Bielke, G., Nieswandt, Z., Wessels, G., Schmarsow, R., Kiefer, H. (1980). Echtzeit-Mammasonographie mit Hilfe eines speziellen Applikators. *Tumordiagnostik 5*:255–259.

Bloomberg, T.J., Chivers, R.C., Price, J.L. (1984). Realtime ultrasonic characteristics of the breast. *Clinical Radiology 35*:21–27.

Calderon, C., Vilkomerson, Mezrich, Etzold, Kingsley, Haskin (1976). Differences in the attenuation of ultrasound by normal, benign, and malignant breast tissue. *Journal of Clinical Ultrasound 4*:249–254.

Carson, P.L., Meyer, C.R., Scherzinger, A.L., Oughton, T.V. (1981). Breast imaging in coronal planes with simultaneous pulse echo and transmission ultrasound. *Science 214*:1141–1143.

Cole-Beuglet, C., Beique, R.A. (1975). Continuous ultrasound B-scanning of palpable breast masses. *Radiology 117*:123–128.

Damascelli, B., Musumeci, R., Orefice, S. (1970). Sonar information about breast tumors. *Radiology 96*:583–586.

Duda, V. (1982). *Ultraschall-Mammographie: Das sonographische Erscheinungsbild anatomischer und pathologischer Strukturen der Mamma unter Anwendung eines Immersionsscanners*. Dissertation, University of Marburg, West Germany, pp. 2–14.

Foster, F.S., Arditi, M., Patterson, M.S., Lee-Chahal, D., Hunt, J.W. (1983). Breast imaging with a conical transducer/annular array hybrid scanner. *Ultrasound in Medicine and Biology 9*:151–164.

Frischbier, H.J. (1985). Empfehlungen zum Einsatz der Mammasonographie. *Deutsches Ärzteblatt 82*:44.

Gros, Ch., Dale, G., Gautherie, M., Gairard, B., Haehnel, P. (1975). Echography-radiography-histology correlation in breast cancer. Excerpta Medica, Amsterdam-Oxford, pp. 253–261.

Harper, P., Kelly-Fry, E. (1980). Ultrasound visualization of the breast in symptomatic patients. *Radiology 137*:465–469.

Howry, D.H., Stott, D.A., Bliss, W.R. (1954). The ultrasonic visualization of carcinoma of the breast and other soft tissue structures. *Cancer 7*:354–358.

Jellins, J., Kossoff, G., Buddee, F.W., Reeve, T.S. (1971). Ultrasonic visualization of the breast. *Medical Journal of Australia 1*:305–307.

Kelly-Fry, E. (1968). A Study of ultrasonic detection of breast disease. First and second quarterly reports to *US pub. Health Serv. Cancer Control Program*, Public Health #6-68193.

Kelly-Fry, E., Harper, P. (1983). Factors critical to highly accurate diagnoses of malignant breast pathologies by ultrasound imaging, In *Ultrasound 82*, Lerski, R.A. and Morley (Eds.), Pergamon Press, New York, 415–421.

Kelly-Fry, E., Jackson, V.P. (1985). Investigations of the advantages of a multiple frequency ultrasound breast examination instrument. In Gill, R.W., Dadd, M.J. (Eds.), *Proc World Federation Ultrasound in Med and Biol*. July 1985:327–328. New York: Pergamon Press.

Kelly-Fry, E., Kossoff, G., Hindman, Jr., H.A. (1972). The potential of ultrasound visualization for detecting the presence of abnormal structures within the female breast. *IEEE Ultrasonics Symposium Proceedings*, pp. 25–30.

Kelly-Fry, E., Sanghvi, N.T., Fry, F.J., Gallager, H.S. (1979). Frequency dependent attenuation of malignant breast tumors studied by the fast fourier transform technique. In Linzer, M. (Ed.): *Ultrasonic Tissue Characterization*, Vol. II. NBS Special Publication 525. *US Government Printing Office, Washington, DC*, 85-91.

Kikuchi, Y., Tanaka, K., Wagai, T. (1957). Early cancer diagnosis through ultrasonics. *Journal of the Acoustical Society of America 29*:824–833.

Kobayashi, T. (1974). Clinical evaluation of ultrasound techniques in breast tumors and malignant abdominal tumors. Excerpta Medica, Amsterdam-Oxford, pp. 191–198.

Kobayashi, T., Nagata, F., Shinoda, A., Nakamura, S., Tanabe, S., Takatani, O. (1977). Ultrasonic diagnosis of early breast cancer: Clinical significance of gray scale expanded echography. *Japanese Journal of Clinical Oncology 7*:55–66.

Kossoff, G., Carpenter, D.A., Radovanovich, G., Robinson, D.E., Garrett, W.J. (1975). Octoson: A new rapid multi-transducer general purpose water-coupling echoscope. Excerpta Medica, Amsterdam-Oxford, pp. 90–95.

Kossoff, G., Garrett, W.J. (1972). Ultrasonic film echography in gynecology and obstetrics. *Australian Journal of Obstetrics and Gynecology 40*:299–305.

Kossoff, G., Kelly-Fry, E., Jellins, J. (1973). Average velocity of ultrasound in the human female breast. *Journal of the Acoustical Society of America 53*: 1730–1736.

Rubin, C.S., Kurtz, A.B., Goldberg, B.B., Feig, S., Cole-Beuglet, C. (1979). Ultrasonic mammographic parenchymal patterns: A preliminary report. *Radiology 130*:515–517.

Wagai, T. (1974). Advances in ultrasonotomography and its clinical evaluation. Excerpta Medica, Amsterdam-Oxford, pp. 186–190.

Wagai, T., Tsutsumi, M. (1977). Ultrasound examination of the breast. In Logan (Ed.), *Breast Carcinoma*, New York, pp. 325–342.

Wells, P.N.T., Evans, K.T. (1968). An immersion scanner for two-dimensional ultrasonic examination of the human breast. *Ultrasonics 6*:220–228.

Wild, J.J., Reid, J.M. (1952). Further pilot echographic studies on the histological structure of tumors of the living intact human breast. *American Journal of Pathology 28*:839–861.

7
The Complementary Role of Blood Flow Assessment to Ultrasonic Imaging

Introduction

Gray-scale ultrasonic imaging has become an accepted clinical modality for displaying the constituent tissues of the breast and providing diagnostic information for the assessment of disease processes (Jellins et al., 1982). Improvements in equipment design, scanning techniques, and display of the ultrasonic characteristic features have resulted in a high degree of accuracy in the interpretation of breast images (Jellins et al., 1985). By utilizing ultrasound to detect vascularity, a functional assessment can be made of the blood flow in the breast. This information, when used in combination with gray-scale imaging, improves overall diagnostic accuracy in assessing patients with breast disease (Jellins et al., 1986).

Ultrasonic Doppler assessment of breast disease was first reported in 1977 (Wells et al., 1977). Different blood flow signals were detected in benign and malignant lesions in a small series of patients examined with a hand-held continuous-wave Doppler probe. Other publications confirmed the presence of specific flow in malignant lesions and concluded that diagnostic information could be obtained to assist in the clinical management of patients with breast disease. Aural interpretation and quantification of Doppler signals enabled a number of characteristic features to be established that differentiated the flow in malignant lesions from the flow existing in the normal vasculature of the breast.

This chapter presents the results of blood flow assessment and ultrasonic imaging on a series of symptomatic patients with benign and malignant lesions. Images were obtained at the Royal North Shore Hospital, New South Wales, Australia, with a four-transducer water-bath scanner. Doppler transducers were incorporated into the water bath so that blood flow assessment could be performed with the patient remaining in the same position for both procedures, thereby ensuring that the Doppler examination was performed on a specific region previously imaged.

Vasculature of the Breast

The breast is a highly vascular organ with an abundant supply of blood originating from three main sources: the internal mammary artery, the lateral thoracic artery, and the intercostal arteries. The contributions from each source vary among individuals but are approximately 50%, 40%, and 10%, respectively. In more detail, the supply comprises

1. Perforating branches of the internal mammary artery arising from the subclavian artery.
2. Mammary branches of the lateral thoracic artery arising from the axillary artery, which is a continuation of the subclavian artery.
3. Intercostal arteries arising from the descending thoracic aorta.

The supply of the whole breast is derived predominantly from the vasculature to the upper quadrants, that is, from the branches of the internal mammary and lateral thoracic arteries (Fig. 7.1). The vascularity to the nipple, areola, and immediate surrounding tissues is complex, resulting from two periareolar anastomotic plexuses located superficially and deep within the parenchyma, both supplied by blood from the three sources previously described.

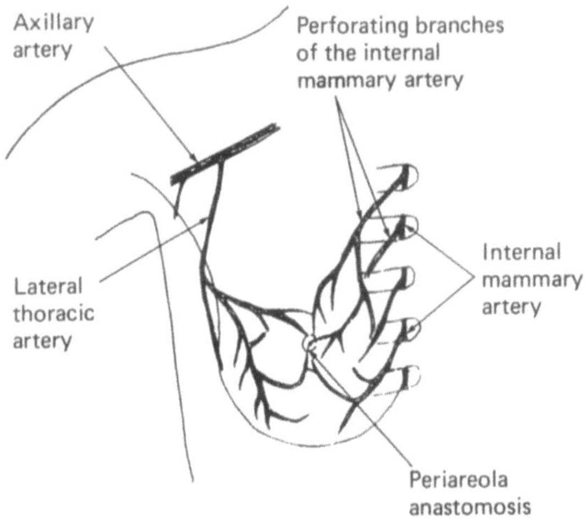

Fig. 7.1. Internal mammary and lateral thoracic arterial supply.

The veins follow the course of the arteries closely and can be divided into superficial and deep vessels. The superficial veins lie under the external layer of the superficial fascia and drain either toward the sternum or upward into the jugular vein. The deep veins consist of the external mammary vein, which empties into the subclavian vein; veins draining into the axillary vein; and intercostal veins draining posteriorly and connecting with the vertebral veins. The link between intercostal and vertebral veins is significant, because it provides the path for breast cancers to metastasize to the central skeletal system (Haagensen, 1971).

While there is considerable variation in the location of vessels among individuals, sufficient vascular symmetry exists between the left and right breasts of each patient to provide a frame of reference for comparison. The vessels are located predominantly in the subcutaneous layers of the breast, varying in depth according to the amount of fatty tissue present. At the periphery of the breast, the perforating branches of the internal mammary artery are situated between 5 mm and 1.0 cm beneath the skin, while the mammary branches of the lateral thoracic artery are located more deeply, normally between 1.0 and 2.5 cm. However, toward the center of the breast, the vessels become more superficial.

Arteries and veins may follow a winding and twisting path in the normal breast, and this can be further altered in the presence of disease (Sakki, 1974). The smaller vessels, arterioles and venules, supply blood to capillary networks, allowing the interchange of physiologic substances between the blood and surrounding tissues. In addition, blood is transferred directly between the arterioles and venules by arteriovenous shunts, without passing through the capillaries (Ganong, 1969; Smith and Kampine, 1984).

Neovascularization

The in situ lesion is the earliest stage at which a malignancy can be detected histologically. At this stage, the lesion is only a few millimeters in diameter and does not possess its own blood supply. It is still avascular, and therefore it does not have the ability to grow beyond a certain volume. In this situation, the lesion is in a dormant state and is relatively harmless.

The potential for growth occurs when the lesion becomes vascularized. Nearby blood vessels send out capillaries, which grow toward the lesion and begin to traverse the center of it. The lesion then has the ability to grow rapidly, because neovascularization provides nutrients and removes waste products at a faster rate than was previously possible.

A vascularized lesion has the ability for exponential growth in comparison with the dormant lesion, which remains constant in size. It compresses, invades, and destroys neighboring tissues. As it grows, the blood supply proliferates, resulting in a multitude of randomly orientated vessels traversing the lesion. With further increase in growth, the vessels concentrate around the periphery of the lesion, resulting in a predominance of blood flow at the advancing edges.

Assessment of Vascularity

Blood flow is not steady but increases and decreases with each cardiac cycle. Pulsatile variations in the velocity of the blood due to systole and diastole are readily demonstrated in the arterial and venous circulation, and have been observed in the arterioles and capillaries surrounding lesions. The flow interrogated during the Doppler examination results from a multitude of vessels, each containing red cells moving at different velocities which contribute different frequency components to the overall Doppler signal (Burns et al., 1982).

The auditory interpretation of the Doppler signal allows the presence of vascularity to be established and provides the basis for recognizing normal flow in arteries and veins. The signals from these vessels are characteristic in sound due to different velocities of the red cells resulting from various parts of the cardiac cycle. In arteries, there are high peak velocities during systole with a rapid decrease in the diastolic phase, in contrast to veins, where the frequencies are lower and the variations between systole and diastole are less pronounced. Since the diameter of veins is greater than that of arteries, lower velocities are present in the venous circulation, and the flow is also modulated by the breathing cycle. Abnormal flow is recognized by the change in the distribution of the velocities during the heart cycle compared with arterial flow, and by the higher amplitude of signals compared with those obtained in the adjacent arteries. The results presented are based on aural interpretation of the Doppler signals.

Contributions from different velocities can be displayed by transforming Doppler signals from the time to the frequency domain. The resultant frequently spectrum is a graph of frequency on the vertical axis as a function of time on the horizontal axis. The intensity at any point is proportional to the amplitude of the signal having that particular frequency. A number of techniques are used to perform the transformation (Kay et al., 1981). The most effective and practical method relies on Fourier analysis, which is implemented conveniently by the fast Fourier transform algorithm. Analyzers using this technique perform the transformation from time to frequency in milliseconds and provide a real-time spectral display (Atkinson and Woodcock, 1982). Frequency spectra of normal and abnormal flow are shown in Figs. 7.2 and 7.3.

The significant features of Doppler signals, in comparison with signals from arterial flow are

1. Higher amplitude.
2. Systolic envelope of increased duration.
3. Increased amplitude during the diastolic phase.

Integration of Flow Assessment with Imaging

The clinical role that can be attributed to the information obtained from the Doppler examination relies on the ability to accurately locate regions that have been previously imaged. In our study, to ensure that blood flow assessment was performed on specific regions within the breast, the Doppler examination was integrated with the imaging examination so that the patient remained in the same position for both procedures. With the Ausonics "System 1" four-transducer water-bath scanner used for this evaluation, plane Doppler transducers with an operating frequency of 10 MHz and a diameter of 1 cm were mounted onto the periphery of one of the imaging transducers so that the sample volume overlapped the focal region of the imaging transducers. The location of the Doppler and imaging transducers relative to the breast is shown in Fig. 7.4. The sample volume of the Doppler transducers measured with a flow phantom is shown in Fig. 7.5. It represents the intensity distribution, whose width is defined by the points where the intensity is 20 dB below the axial value.

Clinical Evaluation

From a series of 538 patients with breast disease who presented at the Royal North Shore Hospital between September 1983 and July 1985, 100 symptomatic patients were examined with the Doppler transducers mounted in the water tank as shown in Fig. 7.6 (Jellins, 1988). The patients were selected for flow assessment on the basis that a palpable lesion was present or a provisional diagnosis could not be made from the information provided by the clinical examination alone.

Flow assessment was performed on patients after completion of the imaging examination. With the patient remaining in the same position for both examinations, the sample volume of the Doppler transducers was located onto the lesion demonstrated on the image. When flow was not detected in a specific location, the imaging transducer was repositioned so that the sample volume interrogated the surrounding tissues. This protocol was repeated until the presence or absence of flow was established. When flow was detected, the same site on the contralateral breast was assessed.

Results

In the series of 100 patients, 71 had benign disease and 29 had malignant disease. The left and right breast of one patient were included separately, and therefore 72 benign examinations are reported

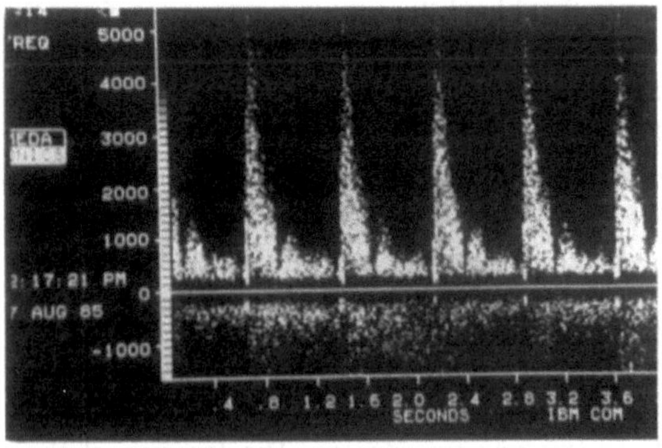

Fig. 7.2. Spectrum analysis of Doppler signals detected from the internal mammary artery. [Reprinted from Jellins, J., Kosoff, G., Reeve, T.S., (1985), with permission.]

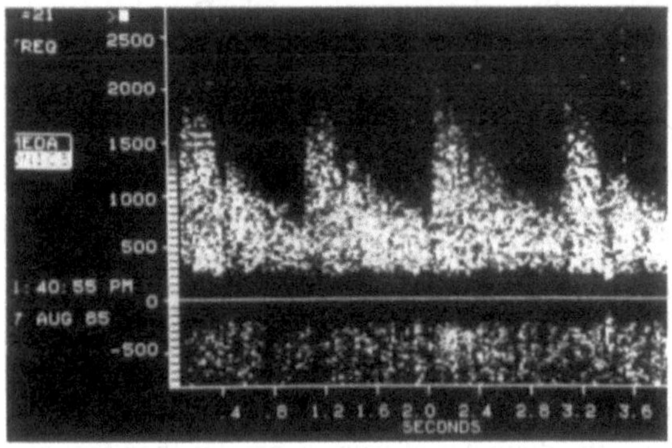

Fig. 7.3. Spectrum analysis of Doppler signals detected from a malignancy. [Reprinted from Jellins, J., Kosoff, G., Reeve, T.S., (1985), with permission.]

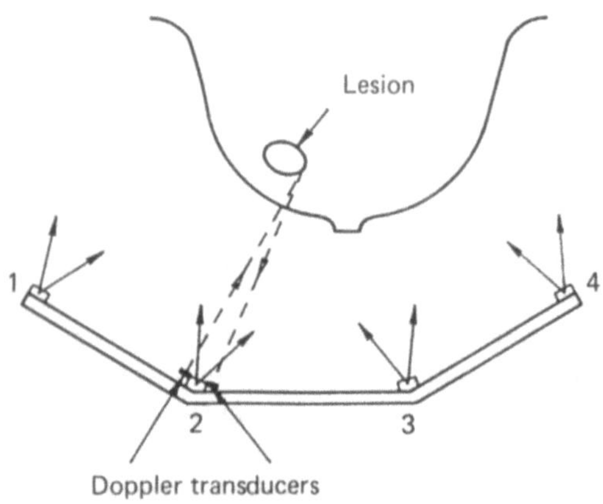

Fig. 7.4. Schematic of the Doppler transducers mounted on the imaging transducer.

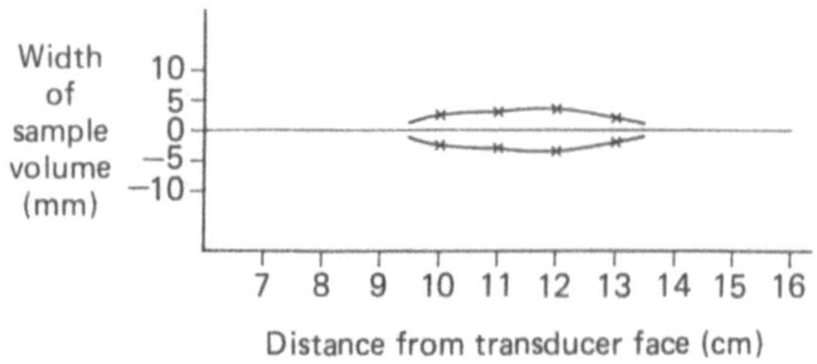

Fig. 7.5. Measured sample volume.

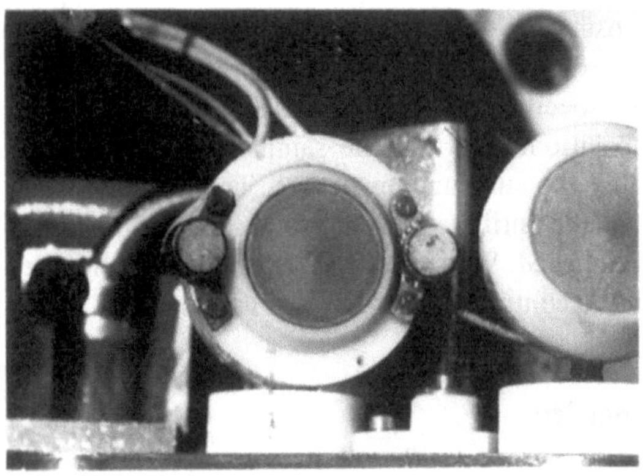

Fig. 7.6. Doppler transducers mounted on the periphery of an imaging transducer.

Table 7.1. Flow assessment in benign conditions.

Benign pathology	Flow assessment	
	Correct	Incorrect
Fibrocystic disease	42	5
Fibroadenoma	4	2
Duct ectasia	3	1
Fatty tissue	2	–
Scar tissue	1	–
Fibrosclerosis	1	2
Abscess	–	1
Fat necrosis	1	–
Fibroadenosis/adenosis	2	1
Lipoma	2	–
Gynecomastia	1	1

Table 7.2. Flow assessment in malignant conditions.

Malignant pathology	Flow assessment	
	Correct	Incorrect
Infiltrating duct carcinoma	24	–
Paget's disease with infiltrating duct carcinoma	1	–
Adenocarcinoma	1	–
Infiltrating papillar carcinoma with cribiform carcinoma	1	–
Intracystic carcinoma	1	–
Diffuse carcinoma in situ	–	1

Table 7.3. Comparison of imaging and flow assessment examinations.

Ultrasonic imaging	Benign pathology		Malignant pathology	
	Doppler correct	Doppler incorrect	Doppler correct	Doppler incorrect
Correct	48	4	26	0
Equivocal	8	4	1	0
Incorrect	3	5	1	1

here. In patients with benign disease, no abnormal flow was detected in 59 examinations, but in 13 Doppler signals consistent with increased vascularity were present. In 28 of the 29 patients with malignant disease, abnormal flow was detected.

The range of benign diseases in the series of patients is listed in Table 7.1. Abnormal flow was detected in five patients with fibrocystic disease. In four of them, biopsy was not performed and the diagnosis was made on the basis that the presenting symptoms remained unchanged over an extended period of time. The one patient biopsied was 72 years of age and the pathology report was benign mammary dysplasia. Of the five patients, one showed a prominence of glandular tissue on imaging with a number of enlarged ducts consistent with benign appearance and another showed dilated ducts and active fibrous and fatty tissue whose appearance was consistent with a benign process, although a malignancy could not be excluded. The three remaining patients on imaging showed lesions whose appearance was consistent with malignancy.

Two patients presented with clinical fibroadenomas which, although benign on imaging, were assessed by Doppler to have abnormal flow. Abnormal blood flow was also detected in the remaining six patients with benign conditions. The images of one patient with duct ectasia were clearly benign in appearance. Three patients had images with equivocal appearances: Two presented with palpable lesions which proved to be, in one case, a hemorrhage with surrounding areas of fibrosclerosis, and in the other case, mammary dysplasia with fibrosclerosis. The remaining patient had an abscess with scar tissue.

In the last two patients with benign disease, malignancies were reported on imaging due to the presence of lesions with jagged edges. The first was a patient with adenotic changes, and the second was a male patient with gynecomastia.

In the patients with malignant disease (Table 7.2), an incorrect flow assessment was obtained in one patient with carcinoma in situ which was not visualized by imaging. Abnormal blood flow was detected in the remaining 28 patients, although in one with an undifferentiated carcinoma lining the cyst wall the imaging report was equivocal, and in another the presence of an infiltrating duct carcinoma was not reported even though malignant features were present.

Discussion

Analysis of the imaging examinations (Table 7.3) shows that the reports were correct for benign disease in 72% (52/72) of the examinations and for malignant disease in 90% (26/29) of the examinations. In the same series, the assessment of blood flow was correct in 82% (59/72) of the examinations in patients with benign disease and 97% (28/29) of those in patients with malignant disease.

The results of imaging and flow assessment can be combined in a number of ways, depending on the emphasis placed on the results of each examination. In this evaluation, the result of ultrasonic imaging was considered to be the prevailing factor in determining the diagnosis. The result of the vascularity assessment was taken into account only when the imaging report was equivocal. Thus, in patients for whom the imaging report was definitive in the diagnosis of the disease (benign or malignant), the result of the Doppler examination was not included in the final assessment. However, when benign or malignant disease was suspected from imaging (equivocal ultrasonic imaging report), the absence or presence of flow was the determining factor in the final report. With this approach, the accuracy for benign disease was 83% (60/72) and for malignant disease was 93% (27/29).

Representative images of breasts for which a discrepancy existed between the pathology report and the results of the imaging and flow assessment examinations are shown in Figs. 7.7 through 7.14.

a

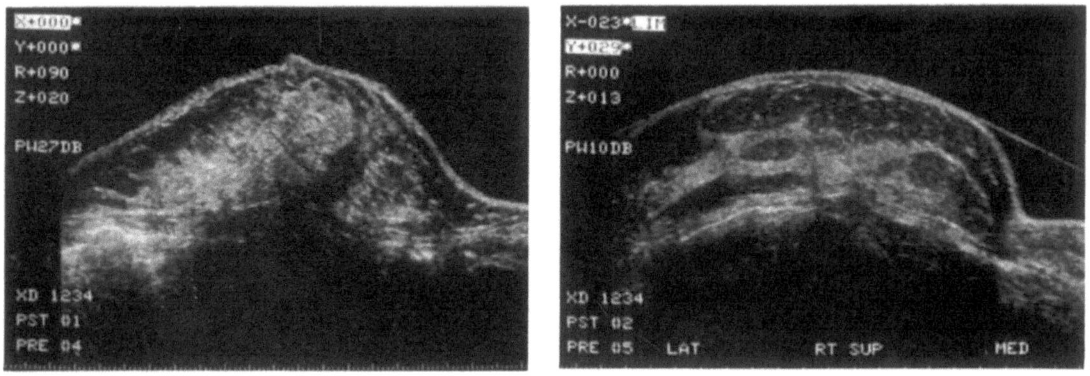

b

Fig. 7.7a,b. Benign pathology. Ultrasonic imaging: equivocal. Doppler examination: correct. **a** Compound parasagittal image of the right breast of a 63-year-old patient who presented with increased nodularity in the breast. The image shows a prominent ductal pattern with general disorganization of the parenchyma in the inferior aspect of the breast. There is no evidence of a discrete lesion, but the prominent ductal pattern caused concern. No abnormal blood flow signals were detected. Biopsy showed benign mammary dysplasia featuring fibrosclerosis and mild ductasia. **b** Compound transverse image of the right breast of a 48-year-old patient who presented with scleroderma and thickening and tenderness lateral to the right nipple. The mammogram showed a distribution of glandular tissue with fatty infiltration. Generalized skin thickening was evident but no lesion was demonstrated. The image shows a well-defined subcutaneous fatty layer with numerous regions of intramammary fat. A 2.5-cm region of low-level echoes was demonstrated medially to the nipple; on biopsy it was found to be fibroadenosis. Examination of the dermis indicated that its appearance was consistent with scleroderma. Doppler signals were not detected.

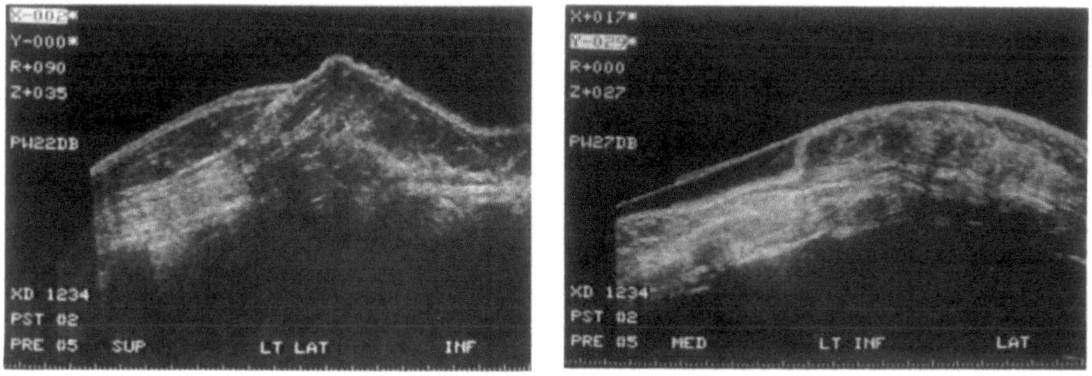

a b

Fig. 7.8a,b. Benign pathology. Ultrasonic imaging: incorrect. Doppler examination: correct. **a** Compound parasagittal image of the left breast of a 55-year-old patient who had a 2.0-cm stage I carcinoma excised 14 months earlier, followed by radiotherapy. The patient presented with a 2-month history of redness and peau d'orange in the upper central area of the breast, suspicious of a recurrent lesion. Mammography 2 months earlier revealed skin thickening, a result of radiotherapy. The ultrasound image shows a 1.2-cm low-level echo lesion 4.0 cm superior to the left nipple. No signals were detected on Doppler examination. Biopsy showed fat necrosis at the operation site and changes due to irradiation with fibrosis and iron pigment granules in the scar tissue. There was no evidence of carcinoma. **b** Compressed compound transverse image of the left breast of a 51-year-old patient who presented with a palpable lump inferior to the nipple. Mammography 1 month earlier revealed an indeterminate increase in density in the lower aspect of the breast. Ultrasonic examination showed a 2.0-cm area of low-level echoes with prominent posterior shadowing in the lower inner quadrant. The features of this lesion were suspicious of malignancy. No Doppler signals were detected in this area. Biopsy revealed the presence of benign mammary dysplasia with evidence of periductal lymphocytic infiltrate.

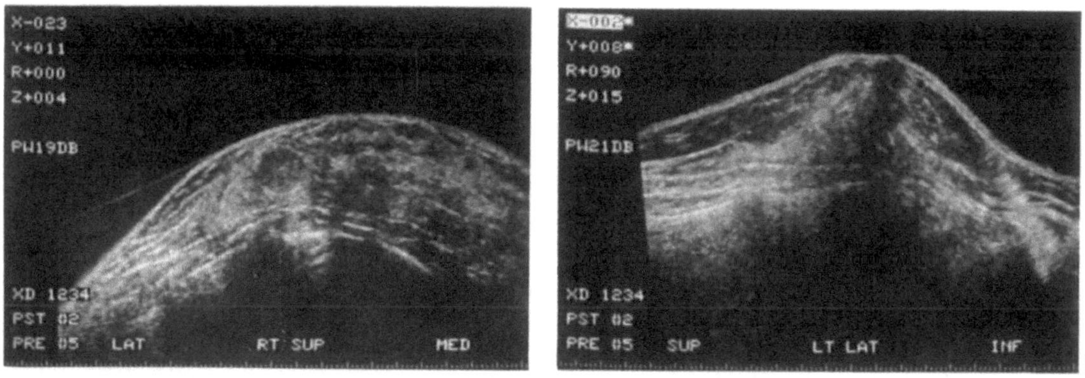

a b

Fig. 7.9a,b. Benign pathology. Ultrasonic imaging: correct. Doppler examination: incorrect. **a** Compound transverse image of the compressed right breast of a 19-year-old patient who at the time of presentation was 9 weeks pregnant. She had a palpable painful lump which had been present for 2 years in the right upper outer quadrant. The image shows a 1.8-cm well-circumscribed lesion with internal echo content and posterior enhancement. The appearance is consistent with a fibroadenoma. Doppler signals of abnormal blood flow were detected in the vicinity of the lesion. However, similar signals were detected in the same region of the contralateral breast. The patient refused surgery. Clinical examination 7 months later showed the condition to be unchanged. **b** Compound parasagittal image of the left breast of a 45-year-old patient who presented with bilateral nipple discharge and flattening of the left nipple of 8 years duration. An X-ray mammogram (xerogram) obtained 5 months previously showed extensive ductal ectasia and calcification but no evidence of a lesion. The image shows a well-defined subcutaneous fatty layer with flattening of the nipple. The central zone of the parenchyma contains predominantly low-level echoes consistent with ductal dilatation and ectasia. Doppler signals characteristic of abnormal blood flow were detected in the central region. Biopsy confirmed the presence of ductal ectasia.

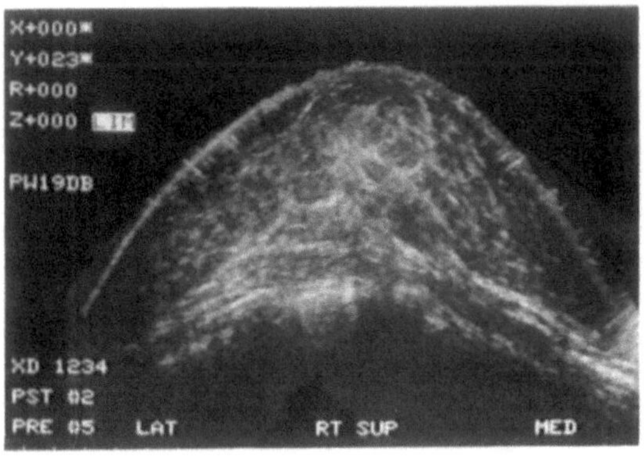

a

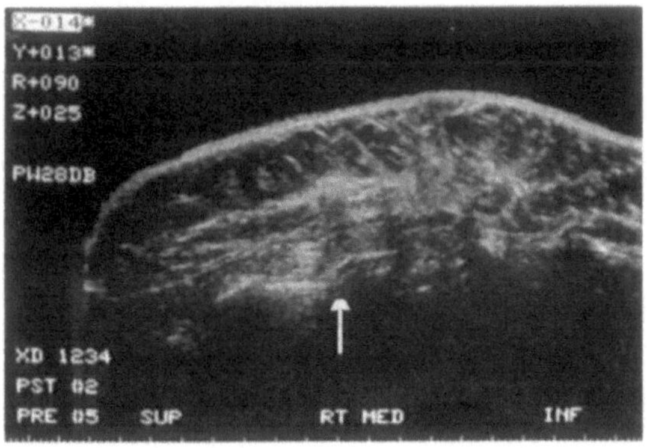

b

Fig. 7.10a,b. Benign pathology. Ultrasonic examination: equivocal. Doppler examination: incorrect. **a** Compound transverse image of the right breast of a 50-year-old patient who presented with a tender palpable lump in the upper inner quadrant together with bruising, resulting from aspiration attempted unsuccessfully 4 days previously. The image shows a pattern of low-level echo areas with ill-defined borders distributed throughout the parenchyma. The overall appearance is consistent with involutional benign changes. Abnormal Doppler signals were detected in the vicinity of the aspiration site. Biopsy of this region showed a 1.0-cm hemorrhage with surrounding areas of fibrosclerosis. **b** Compound parasagittal image of the right breast of a 62-year-old patient who presented with a palpable lump superior to the nipple. Nine months previously the patient had a biopsy for fibrosclerosis with focal sclerosis adenosis, but the present lump was superior to the scar. The image shows an area of disruption (arrow) consistent with a benign process. Doppler signals consistent with abnormal blood flow were detected in the vicinity of the palpable lump. Mammography 1 month following the examination identified a lesion in one projection, but its nature was uncertain and its appearance had not changed since a previous mammographic examination 1 year earlier. Biopsy showed benign mammary dysplasia with fibrosclerosis and focal sclerosing adenosis.

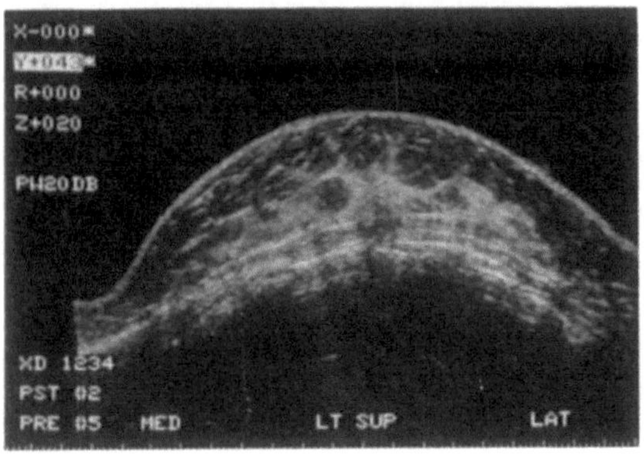

a

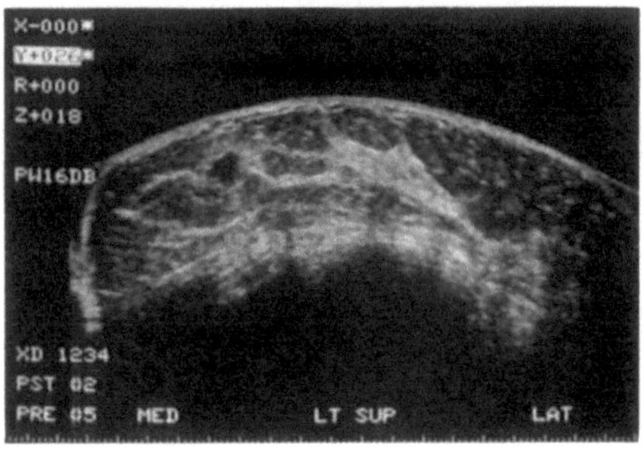

b

Fig. 7.11a,b. Benign pathology. Ultrasonic imaging: incorrect. Doppler examination: incorrect. **a** Compound transverse image of the left breast of a 62-year-old patient who had a carcinoma removed 2 years previously from the right breast. One year later an ultrasonic examination displayed a lesion 4.0 cm above the nipple. The current examination showed that the lesion had remained unchanged. The image shows a 2.0-cm lesion with equivocal characteristics; because of the patient's age and clinical history, a malignancy cannot be excluded. Doppler signals indicating abnormal blood flow were detected. The unchanged appearance of the lesion between the two examinations indicated that the lesion was benign and therefore no surgical procedure was instigated. **b** Compound transverse image of the compressed left breast of a 72-year-old patient who presented with a palpable lump in the upper inner quadrant. The image shows a well-defined 1.0-cm area with no internal echoes. The borders are jagged and there is an increase in the number of echoes anterior to the lesion in the subcutaneous fat layer. The appearance is consistent with a malignancy. Doppler signals indicated abnormal blood flow. Biopsy proved this to be benign mammary dysplasia.

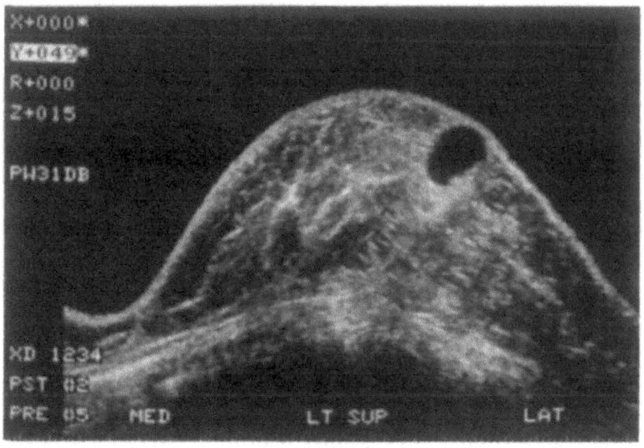

Fig. 7.12. Malignant pathology. Ultrasonic imaging: equivocal. Doppler examination: correct. Compound transverse image of the left breast of a 56-year-old patient who presented with a tender lump in the upper outer quadrant. A fine-needle aspiration biopsy sample obtained 1 week previously contained cells suspicious of malignancy. The image shows a 2.2-cm liquid-filled lesion with moderate intracystic proliferation on the posterolateral margin. Abnormal Doppler signals characteristic of a malignancy were detected in the vicinity of the lesion. Excision biopsy demonstrated an undifferentiated carcinoma lining the cyst with some degree of infiltration into the surrounding subcutaneous and parenchymal tissues.

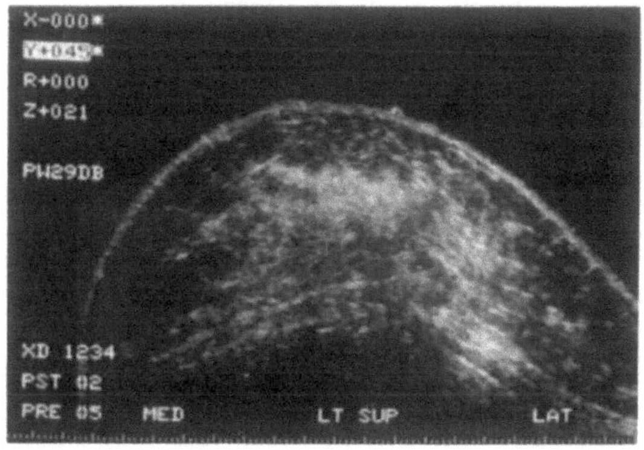

Fig. 7.13. Malignant pathology. Ultrasonic imaging: incorrect. Doppler examination: correct. Compound transverse image of the left breast of a 64-year-old patient who presented with a palpable lesion in the left axilla. The image, taken at a level 4.5 cm above the nipple, shows a 1.0 × 2.4-cm area of parenchymal disruption in the lateral aspect of the breast. Because no discrete lesion was demonstrated, the report did not specify the presence of a malignancy, even though both primary and secondary ultrasonic features were present. Doppler signals indicated abnormal blood flow. Biopsy confirmed the presence of a 2.0-cm infiltrating duct carcinoma.

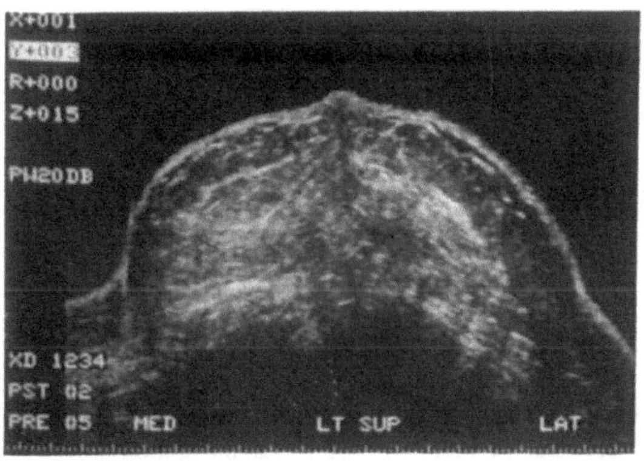

Fig. 7.14. Malignant pathology. Ultrasonic imaging: incorrect. Doppler examination: incorrect. Compound transverse image of the left breast of a 65-year-old patient who presented with a nipple discharge. The image shows a number of enlarged ducts within and posterior to the nipple region. The remainder of the breast contains a well-demarcated subcutaneous fatty layer with involutional changes in the mammary layer. No discrete lesion could be demonstrated in the images. Doppler signals were not detected in the vicinity of the nipple and adjacent areas. Pathology revealed the presence of diffuse carcinoma in situ.

Conclusions

The diagnostic accuracy of ultrasonic imaging alone in the differentiation of benign and malignant lesions appears to have reached an upper limit. This limit can be improved by including the results of tissue vascularity assessment. Combining the Doppler examination with imaging increases the accuracy of diagnosis of breast disease by reducing the number of false-positive and -negative reports obtained with imaging. In 100 symptomatic patients, the 20 false-positive and 3 false-negative reports from imaging alone decreased to 12 and 2 respectively, when the results of both examination procedures were combined.

Bibliography

Anson, B.J., Wright, R.R. (1939). Blood supply of the mammary gland. *Surgery, Gynecology, and Obstetrics* *69*:468.

Atkinson, P., Woodcock, J.P. (1982). *Doppler Ultrasound and Its Use in Clinical Measurement*. Academic Press, London.

Bamber, J.C., Sambrook, M., Minasian, H., Hill, C.R. (1983). Doppler study of blood flow in breast cancer. In Jellins and Kobayashi (Eds.), *Ultrasonic Examination of the Breast*. John Wiley, Chichester, England, p. 371.

Boyd, J., Jellins, J., Kossoff, G., Reeve, T.S. (1985). Combined B-mode and Doppler examinations of the breast. In Gill and Dadd (Eds.), *WFUMB '85 Proceedings*. Pergamon Press, Sydney, Australia, p. 365.

Burns, P.N., Halliwell, M., Webb, A.J., Wells, P.N.T. (1982). Ultrasonic Doppler studies of the breast. *Ultrasound in Medicine and Biology 8*:127.

Burns, P.N., Virjee, J.M., Gowland, M., Rimmer, S., Wells, P.N.T. (1983). The origin of Doppler shift signals from breast tumours. In Jellins and Kobayashi (Eds.), *Ultrasonic Examination of the Breast*. John Wiley, Chichester, England, p. 379.

Folkman, J. (1974). Tumour angiogenesis. *Advances in Cancer Research 19*:331.

Folkman, J. (May 1976). The vascularization of tumours. *Scientific American*, p. 59.

Gallager, H.S., Leis, H.P., Snyderman, R.K., Urban, J.A. (Eds.) (1978). *The Breast*. C.V. Mosby, St. Louis, MO.

Ganong, W.F. (1969). Dynamics of blood and lymph flow. In *Review of Medical Physiology*. Lange Medical Publications, Los Altos, CA, p. 458.

Gros, Ch.M., Dale, G., Gairand, B. (1978). Breast echography: Criteria of malignancy and results. In Kurjak (Ed.), *Recent Advances in Ultrasound Diagnosis*. Excerpta Medica, Amsterdam, p. 292.

Haagensen, C.D. (1971). *Diseases of the Breast*. W.B. Saunders, Philadelphia. p. 27.

Jellins, J. (1985). B-mode and Doppler assessment of breast disease. In Jellins, Kossoff, and Croll (Eds.), *Proceedings of the Fourth International Congress on the Ultrasonic Examination of the Breast*. Sydney, Australia, p. 215.

Jellins, J. (1988). Combining imaging and vascularity assessment of breast lesions. Submitted to Ultrasound in Medicine and Biology.

Jellins, J., Boyd, J., Kossoff, G., Reeve, T.S. (1985). Primary and secondary features of solid breast lesions. In Gill and Dadd (Eds.), *WFUMB '85 Proceedings*, Pergamon Press, Sydney, Australia, p. 330.

Jellins, J., Kossoff, G., Boyd, J., Reeve, T.S. (1983). The complementary role of Doppler to the B-mode examination of the breast. *Journal of Ultrasound in Medicine 2* (No. 10):29.

Jellins, J., Kossoff, G., Greenleaf, J.F., Bahn, R.C. (1986). Breast tissue characterization. In Greenleaf (Ed.), *Tissue Characterization with Ultrasound* (Vol. 11). CRC Press, Boca Raton, FL, p. 95.

Jellins, J., Kossoff, G., Reeve, T.S. (1985). Ultrasonic imaging of small breast lesions: The potential for screening. In Rossotto, Durante, Belcastro, and Santini (Eds.), *Attualità in Endocrinochirurgia*. Monduzzi Editore S.P.A., Bologne, Italy. p. 373.

Jellins, J., Reeve, T.S., Croll, J., Kossoff, G. (1982). Results of breast echography examinations in Sydney, Australia 1972–1979. *Seminars in Ultrasound*. Grune and Stratton, New York, p. 58.

Kay, D.M., Marple, S.M. (1981). Spectrum analysis – a modern perspective. *Proceedings of the IEEE 69*(No. 11):1380.

Lypacewicz, G., Powalowski, T., Lukawska, K. (1978). Ultrasonic examination of breast tumours with Doppler method. In Filipczynski and Zieniuk (Eds.), *Proceedings of the Second Congress of the Federation of Acoustical Societies of Europe* (Vol. 2). Polish Academy of Sciences, Warsaw, p. 153.

Maliniac, J.W. (1943). Arterial blood supply of the breast. *Archives of Surgery 47*:329.

Minasian, H., Bamber, J.C. (1982). A preliminary assessment of an ultrasonic Doppler method for the study of blood flow in human breast cancer. *Ultrasound in Medicine and Biology 8*:357.

Netter, F.H., Geschickter, C.F. (1965). Anatomy and pathology of the mammary gland. In Netter (Ed.), *The Ciba Collection of Medical Illustrations Vol. 2: Reproductive System*. Ciba Pharmaceutical Company, Summit, N.J., p. 245.

Sakki, S. (1974). Angiography of the female breast. Department of Diagnostic Radiology, University of Oulu, Oulu, Sweden.

Smith, J.J., Kampine, J.P. (1984). *Circulatory Physiology–The Essentials*. Williams and Wilkins, Baltimore.

Warren, B.A. (1979). The vascular morphology of tumours. In Peterson (Ed.), *Tumour Blood Circulation*. CRC Press, Boca Raton, FL, p. 1.

Wells, P.N.T., Halliwell, M., Skidmore, R., Webb, A.J., Woodcock, J.P. (1977). Tumour detection by ultrasonic Doppler blood flow signals. *Ultrasonics 15*:231.

White, D.M., Cledgett, P.R. (1978). Breast carcinoma detection by ultrasonic Doppler signals. *Ultrasound in Medicine and Biology 4*:329.

Index

MIX
Papier aus verantwortungsvollen Quellen
Paper from responsible sources
FSC® C105338

If you have any concerns about our products,
you can contact us on
ProductSafety@springernature.com

In case Publisher is established outside the EU,
the EU authorized representative is:
Springer Nature Customer Service Center GmbH
Europaplatz 3, 69115 Heidelberg, Germany

Printed by Libri Plureos GmbH
in Hamburg, Germany